The Keto Crock Pot Cookbook

Quick And Easy Ketogenic Crock Pot Recipes For Smart People

Table Of Contents

Introduction

Greetings! Thanks for joining us here at, "The Keto Crock Pot Cookbook."

This is a book especially for people who have taken the Ketogenic Diet under their wing, and who want to put their Crock Pot to good use.

Perhaps you have recently purchased your first Crock Pot and are looking for some ideas and inspiration for Crock Pot-friendly Ketogenic recipes? In that case, you've come to right place, and I hope you find some great ideas!

I am a total food lover, Keto dieter, and Crock Pot user. I am not a nutritionist, professional chef, or doctor. However, I *am* a great cook and recipe creator, with a thorough working knowledge of the Ketogenic Diet. I have compiled the information in this book based on my understanding, and have attempted to word it in a user-friendly way! There's lots of science and "complicated stuff" involved in the Ketogenic Diet, but I have aimed to provide the need-to-know information in a practical and useful way. There are so many great sources online if you want to explore the more complicated side of the diet!

The recipes in this book are simple, adaptable, Keto-friendly, and easy to create in your Crock Pot. You will find recipes for appetizers, breakfast, soups & stews, meat, seafood, and dessert!

Go forth, have fun, and let's cook together!

Chapter 1: The Ketogenic diet

What is the Ketogenic diet?

The Ketogenic Diet is a low-carb diet which nudges the body into a metabolic state called "Ketosis". When you reach Ketosis, your body starts to produce Ketones, which are used as an energy source. The Ketogenic diet relies heavily on the correct intake of macronutrients (carbs, fats, proteins) - very low carb, high fat, and moderate protein.

Here is a rundown of how the Ketogenic diet works inside your body (in layman's terms!): when you eat carbs, your body uses them as its first source of energy. This includes all starches, sugars (including the sugars in fruit!) and grains. This means that the fat you consume is stored away and is not used as energy. When you deprive your body of carbs, something pretty amazing happens. First, your body will find energy by using stored-up glycogen (glycogen is what carbs are converted to before they are stored in your body). Once the glycogen has been used up and the carb-flow has run dry, your body turns to stored fats to use as energy. Once stored fats are being used as the primary energy source, your liver gets the message to start producing Ketones to be used as an extra energy hit. When this happens...woohoo, you've reached ketosis!

I won't bore you with more picky details, as I'm sure you've read up on the Ketogenic diet enough already. Let's get on to the important stuff, what you can and can't eat!

What you can eat

The Ketogenic diet is very strict when it comes to what you are allowed to munch on. If you eat the wrong things (i.e. carbs and sugars), then Ketosis is ruined and you must start again. It sounds strict and cumbersome, but it's actually easier than you might think. Here are the foods you are allowed to eat:

Non-starchy vegetables

Choose vegetables that grow above ground. Dark, leafy greens are the best choices as they are very low in carbohydrates and are packed with nutrients. Fill your meals with these veggies:

Spinach

- Kale
- Chard
- Lettuce
- Green capsicums
- Broccoli
- Cauliflower
- Mushrooms
- Green beans
- Cabbage
- Tomatoes
- Eggplant

Berries

Berries are the only fruits you can eat on the Ketogenic diet. Eat small amounts of these berries:

- Raspberries
- Strawberries (eat very sparingly)
- Blackberries

Meat

Incorporate moderate amounts of meat into your diet, to provide you with protein and iron. Because protein must be eaten in moderation, smaller portions of meat are ideal. Choose these meats:

Bacon

- Minced lamb
- Minced beef
- Chicken thigh
- Chicken breast (eat small amounts as it's quite high in protein)
- Lamb leg
- Roast beef
- Whole roast chicken

Seafood

Fish and seafood are great choices to provide you with fats, oils, and moderate protein. Choose these fishy creatures:

- Fresh salmon
- Oily white fish
- Shellfish
- Tinned tuna
- Tinned salmon

Dairy

Dairy products are allowed on Keto, as long as they are full-fat, unsweetened, and low carb. Milk is not recommended on the Ketogenic diet, so stick with cream instead. Choose these dairy products:

- Full-fat cream
- Full-fat unsweetened Greek yogurt
- Cream cheese
- Sour cream
- Soft cheeses (brie, mozzarella)
- Hard cheeses (cheddar, parmesan)

Nuts and seeds

Nuts and seeds are allowed on the Ketogenic diet, as long as they are eaten in moderation. They are great as snacks and sprinkles to add healthy fats and yummy texture. Choose these lower-carb nuts and seeds:

- Macadamia nuts
- Pecans
- Brazil nuts
- Walnuts
- Almonds
- Hazelnuts
- Pine nuts
- Chia seeds
- Flax seeds
- Pumpkin seeds

Oils and dressings

Oils and fats which are categorized as "saturated" and "monounsaturated" are the best options to choose for dressings and cooking. These include:

- Butter
- Olive oil
- Coconut oil
- Avocado oil

Alcohol

You can drink alcohol on the Keto diet as long as you are very careful about what you drink, and how much. When you first start Keto, I recommend that you completely cut alcohol from your diet while your body gets used to the change. After a few weeks, you could incorporate small amounts of low-carb alcohol such as plain vodka. Check the labels on wine bottles to make sure you aren't purchasing a carbo-loaded, sugar-laden tipple! A small glass of low-carb wine won't harm your Keto efforts, just be sure to limit yourself to a glass or 2. Using wine in your cooking is fine, as once it has been spread between a few servings, the amount you consume is very little.

Sweeteners

As you will soon see in the dessert section of this book, you can use natural, non-sugar sweeteners in your desserts. I opt for liquid stevia, as I think it offers the best taste!

What you can't eat

The "can't" list is strict, yes, but I shall keep it short and sweet. Instead of going through each item you can't eat, it's easier to outline the entire food group so you know what kinds of food to avoid. Basically, if it's starchy, grainy, fruity, or sweet…it's out of bounds!

Fruits

Fruits are full of carbs and sugars. You must completely avoid most fruits, (apart from a few berries). A very small amount of citrus juice (lemon, lime, orange) used as a flavoring is fine.

Grains

No grains allowed! This includes all wheat products. Breads, baked goods, cereals, corn products, rice and rice products, quinoa and quinoa products are all to be avoided! Basically, if it's starchy, grainy, and screams "carbs" – keep well away.

Starchy vegetables

Potatoes, sweet potatoes, and yams are to be crossed of your shopping list. They are full of carbs and must be eliminated from your diet. A very small amount of carrots and parsnips are permitted, (but I think it's best to avoid them completely, just to be safe).

Sugar

Sweets, ice cream, cakes...you know the drill. Anything sweet or sugary is a major no-no. This includes honey! Use stevia to sweeten your dishes if need be.

Benefits of the Ketogenic diet

The Ketogenic diet is very beneficial for a number of reasons! In fact, the diet was originally formulated to help people with epilepsy to manage their symptoms. Some people choose to live a Ketogenic lifestyle for weight loss reasons, or simply to live a healthier life with decreased risk of disease. Here are some of the amazing benefits of the Ketogenic diet:

Weight loss

By nudging your body into using stored fat as energy, you can look forward to a more trim and healthy body! By cutting out carbs and sugars, you will naturally be cutting out many high-calorie foods such as cakes, fried starches, and sweets. By swapping these foods for more vegetables and healthy fats, your calorie intake will drop, helping you to drop weight!

Reduced risk of diseases

The Ketogenic diet helps to fight against diseases such as Type 2 Diabetes, metabolic disease, obesity, heart disease, and many more. The Ketogenic diet encourages higher levels of "good cholesterol" and lower levels of "bad cholesterol" which is great news for your heart. The increased intake of nutrients in your diet helps to keep your body strong and healthy.

Increased energy

By cutting out those sugary and starchy foods, you will be doing your blood sugar levels a favor! Sugary foods spike our blood sugar, causing major highs and lows in our energy levels. Eating foods which release energy slowly and steady will help you to remain focused and strong throughout the day.

Reduced belly fat

Losing weight and losing belly fat isn't always the same thing! It can be very hard to lose that annoying fat around our middle. The Ketogenic diet can really help to shift the fat that likes to roll up when we sit down! What's more, Keto can help to remove the fat we *can't* see: visceral fat which hides around our vital organs. By losing fat around our middle, we are decreasing our chances of developing certain diseases, and keeping our organs safe and healthy.

Decreased cravings (after a while)

Sugar and starch cravings can be very powerful and irresistible! The thing is, the more sugar and starch you eat...the more you crave it. Once you cut these foods out of your diet and have allowed your body to get used to new energy sources, the cravings tend to disappear. Not *thinking* about "bad" foods is the best way to keep yourself from *eating* those foods. This is one of the best benefits of the Ketogenic diet; by changing your tastes and habits, you can change your lifestyle and enjoy a healthy and energetic life.

Chapter 2: Crock Pot

What is a Crock Pot?

Well, this can be a tricky question. Many people use the term "crock pot" to refer to a slow cooker, regardless of the brand or make. In fact, there is an official "Crock Pot", which is the slow cooker we will be using and referring to in this book.

When talking about slow cookers in general, I would describe them as a "one-pot" appliance which allows the user to cook dishes slowly and without need for supervision. The Crock Pot is most commonly known for slow-cooked meat dishes, stews, and soups, due to the long cook time and even heat distribution.

How to use the Crock Pot

The Crock Pot is incredibly easy to use! That's part of the major appeal of this genius appliance. There are not many ways you can mess up your food with the Crock Pots, but there are some tips to follow to ensure a successful result!

Temperature

Most Crock Pot models have a LOW and HIGH setting. You need to adjust your cooking time according to the temperature setting. For example, if you have the HIGH setting on, your dish might take 4 hours to cook, but if you have the LOW setting on, it might take 8 hours. Follow the guidelines in your Crock Pot handbook, and stick to the time suggestions in these recipes (and others!).

Size and servings

When purchasing your Crock Pot, choose a size that suits your regular serving needs; i.e. if you have a family of 5, choose a large pot. The thing is, you should never over-fill the Crock Pot. If you add too many ingredients, the food won't cook evenly, and it might turn out sloppy and flavorless. Don't fill the Crock Pot more than two thirds full and you'll be fine!

Time

If you'd like to cook your meal throughout the day, while you are out and about, you can do so! Choose a LOW setting and cook the meal slowly, for at least 8 hours (or according to the recipe instructions). When the meal has finished cooking, the Crock Pot will automatically switch to WARM until you are ready to devour your meal.

Liquids

Crock Pots and slow cookers do not reduce liquids. When you are cooking in a regular pot or pan, the liquid you add will evaporate, thicken, and reduce: this does not happen when cooking with the Crock Pot! The liquid you add at the start will be there at the end. Therefore, be careful with the amount of liquid you are adding to your dish. You can reduce and simmer liquids such as wine and cream in a pot or frypan before you add it to the slow cooker. When using a recipe made especially for a Crock Pot or slow cooker, follow it carefully and you'll be perfectly fine.

What are the benefits of using the Crock Pot?

Anyone who owns and uses a Crock Pot will rave to you about the many benefits of this appliance! Here are some of the fantastic reasons to incorporate the Crock Pot into your cooking routine:

Convenience

Instead of hauling out an armful of pots and pans from the cupboards, just use the Crock Pot! It's already there on the bench, so load it up. All you need to do is clean the inner pot after you're done, and put it back into the Crock Pot unit, ready for next time.

Ready-to-go meals

A crazy lifestyle doesn't mean that you need to sacrifice wholesome and delicious meals. The amazing thing about the Crock Pot is that you can leave it to cook your meal while you are at work, or even overnight. Load the ingredients into the pot, set the temperature and time, and walk away.

Tender meat

Slow cooked meat is tender, melt-in-the-mouth, and satisfying. You can achieve this by simply throwing the meat into the pot with any flavorings you like, a small amount of liquid, and simply forget about it for hours while you live your life!

Versatility

As you will see in the recipe section, you can cook anything in the Crock Pot! Meat, vegetables, seafood, dessert, starters! You can cook your dish entirely in the Crock Pot, from start to finish, or you can finish it off in a hot fry pan to give a golden crunch to meat and veggie dishes.

Chapter 3: Ketogenic recipes

Notes on these recipes

All of these recipes comply with the Ketogenic diet, and are packed with nutritious and tasty ingredients. The oil I have chosen to use in each recipe is olive oil, but you can substitute for coconut oil if you prefer. The approximate times I have supplied for each recipe refer to the cook time only. However, most of these recipes are very quick to prepare, so you only need to add another ten minutes or so to get the total time!

These recipes work in any slow cooker. Whether or not your slow cooker is a genuine Crock Pot, or another brand, it doesn't matter! These recipes will work in any model.

Appetizers

Appetizers don't need to be fiddly or time consuming. These recipes are totally Keto-friendly, and can be made partially or entirely in your Crock Pot or slow cooker. If you want to make these recipes to eat as a light main course instead of a starter, simply adjust the quantities and make as much as you require.

Garlic and chili Brussel's sprouts with spicy mayo dip

Brussel's sprouts are full of nutritional value and flavor. I don't think they deserve their terrible reputation! These Brussel's sprouts are served with a creamy and spicy mayo dip, ideal for a starter or appetizer.

Serves: 6 as a starter
Time: approximately 2 hours and 10 minutes

Ingredients:
- 12 – 16 Brussel's sprouts
- 3 garlic cloves, crushed
- 1 tsp dried chili flakes
- ½ cup egg-based mayonnaise
- ½ tsp cayenne pepper
- ½ lemon

Method:
1. Drizzle some olive oil into a skillet and heat.
2. Once the oil is hot, add the Brussel's sprouts and toss in the hot oil for about 1 minute, until golden on the outside.
3. Place the sprouts into the Crock Pot and sprinkle the crushed garlic, chili flakes, salt, and pepper over the top.
4. Place the lid onto the Crock Pot and set the temperature to LOW.
5. Leave for 2 hours, turning once after 1 hour.
6. In a small bowl, mix together the mayonnaise, cayenne pepper, and the juice of half a lemon.
7. Remove the sprouts from the crock pot and serve on a platter with the spicy mayonnaise dip.

Chicken, bacon, and cheddar taste teasers

These are called "teasers" because they are small, bite-sized pieces which are ideal as a starter or appetizer. Be careful...once you have one, you'll want the whole lot!

Serves: 6 as a starter
Time: approximately 4 hours

Ingredients:
- 2 large chicken breasts, each cut into 6 pieces
- 1/2 cup cheddar cheese, grated
- 4 garlic cloves, crushed
- 6 slices of streaky bacon, each cut in half width ways

Method:
1. Lightly coat the Crock Pot with olive oil.
2. Wrap each piece of chicken with bacon.
3. Add the bacon-wrapped chicken pieces to the Crock Pot, sprinkle with salt, pepper, and crushed garlic.
4. Place the lid onto the pot and set the temperature to LOW.
5. Leave to cook for 4 hours.
6. Once the chicken pieces are cooked, remove from the Crock Pot and place in an oven-proof dish.
7. Preheat the oven to 180 degrees Celsius, (356 Fahrenheit).
8. Sprinkle the chicken dish with cheese and place in the oven until the cheese has melted.
9. Remove from the oven and serve while hot.

Pork and chive meatballs

Meatballs on toothpicks, what could be a simpler starter? I like to serve these with a spicy tomato sauce, or a lemon aioli. You can use any kind of minced meat you like if you don't feel like using pork.

Serves: 6 as a starter
Time: approximately 4 hours

Ingredients:
- 1 lb minced pork
- 1 egg
- 2 garlic cloves, crushed
- ¼ cup ground almonds
- 2 tbsp finely chopped chives

Method:
1. In a large bowl, mix together the pork, egg, garlic, ground almonds, chives, salt, and pepper until combined.
2. Roll the mixture into about 18 balls.
3. Drizzle the Crock Pot with olive oil.
4. Lay the meatballs into the crock pot and drizzle with olive oil.
5. Place the lid onto the pot and set the timer to LOW.
6. Cook for 4 hours.
7. Once the meatballs are cooked, take them out of the pot and serve on a serving platter with a small bowl of toothpicks.

Salmon-wrapped double cheese bites

I know, this recipe sounds completely over the top! Salmon wrapped around TWO types of cheese? Yes. These delicious little starters are so rich you only need one or two. I like to finely zest a lemon over the top of the bites before serving, as it provides a lovely freshness.

Serves: 6 - 8 as a starter
Time: approximately 2 hours

Ingredients:
- 4 strips of smoked salmon, (approximately 50gm) cut in half lengthways
- ¼ lb firm cream cheese, cut into 8 chunks
- ¼ lb mozzarella cheese, cut into 8 chunks
- 1 spring onion, finely chopped
- 1 lemon

Method:
1. Take one piece of cream cheese and one piece of mozzarella, press them together and sprinkle with a small amount of spring onion.
2. Wrap the cheese bundle in smoked salmon.
3. Repeat this process until all of the ingredients have been used, there should be 8 pieces.
4. Drizzle some oil into the Crock Pot and place the salmon bites in one layer into the pot.
5. Place the lid onto the pot at set the temperature at LOW.
6. Leave to cook for 2 hours.
7. Once the bites are cooked, finely grate the zest of half a lemon over them and place on a serving platter.

Mini lamb and eggplant skewers with yogurt dip

Lamb, eggplant, and yoghurt go together so incredibly well. These skewers are a fantastic starter or side dish for a Summer barbeque. If you don't have minced lamb, you can certainly replace with any other meat you like. This recipe makes 4 skewers, with the idea that each person has 1 skewer as a starter. You can double the recipe to serve more people if you wish.

Serves: 4 as a starter
Time: approximately 4 hours

Ingredients:
- 1 lb minced lamb
- 2 garlic cloves, crushed
- 1 egg, lightly beaten
- 1 lemon
- 1 large eggplant, cut into 12 even chunks
- ¾ cup full-fat Greek yoghurt
- 2 tbsp fresh mint leaves, finely chopped

Method:
1. In a medium-sized bowl, mix together the minced lamb, garlic cloves, egg, salt, pepper, and zest of one lemon.
2. Roll the lamb mixture into 12 balls.
3. Place the eggplant chunks on a damp tea towel and sprinkle them with salt and leave while you prepare the yoghurt dip in advance.
4. Mix together the yoghurt, fresh mint, and juice of the lemon in a small bowl, cover and store in the fridge until needed.
5. Rub the eggplant chunks with olive oil.
6. Take 4 skewers and "fill" them with alternating lamb mince balls and eggplant chunks, so that each skewer has 3 lamb mince balls and 3 eggplant chunks.
7. Drizzle some olive oil into the Crock Pot.
8. Lay the skewers into the Crock Pot and set the temperature at LOW.
9. Cook for 4 hours, turning once, after the 2-hour mark.
10. Remove the skewers from the pot and serve on a platter with the yoghurt dip.

Zucchini, beef, feta, and almond parcels

For this recipe, we call on zucchini to be a stand-in for pastry! Strips of zucchini encase salty feta cheese, crunchy almonds, and tender minced beef. Like all of these recipes, use your favorite minced meat if beef isn't preferable!

Serves: 6 as a starter
Time: approximately 4 hours

Ingredients:
- 1 lb minced beef
- 1 egg, lightly beaten
- 2 garlic cloves, crushed
- 2 large zucchinis, peeled into strips with a peeler
- ¼ pound cup firm feta cheese, cut into small chunks
- 1/4 cup slivered almonds, roughly chopped

Method:
1. In a medium-sized bowl, mix together the minced beef, egg, garlic, salt, and pepper.
2. Take a chunk of feta cheese and "coat" it in the beef mixture, so it resembles a roughly-shaped meatball, the feta shouldn't be visible as it should be entirely cased in beef mince.
3. Roll the filled beef mince ball in the chopped almonds until roughly coated.
4. Tightly wrap each almond-coated meatball in a strip of zucchini, place a tooth pick through the center to keep it all together if you wish.
5. Drizzle some olive oil into the Crock Pot.
6. Lay the zucchini/beef parcels along the bottom of the pot, rubbing them in the oil to prevent them from sticking.
7. Place the lid onto the pot and set the temperature at LOW.
8. Cook for 4 hours, turning once, after the 2-hour mark.
9. Remove from the pot and serve on a platter with any dip you like, garlic yoghurt would be lovely!

Spiced macadamia and chicken nibbles

Macadamia nuts are such a glorious way to crumb chicken, as they are so crunchy and give a slightly creamy flavor. The mixture of spices really makes this starter an exciting beginning to a dinner party or meal.

Serves: 6 – 8 as a starter
Time: approximately 4 hours

Ingredients:
- 1.5 lb chicken nibbles
- 2 eggs, lightly beaten
- ½ cup salted, roasted macadamia nuts, finely chopped
- 2 tsp mixed paprika, chili powder, ground cumin, ground coriander

Method:
1. Mix the chopped macadamia nuts with the mixed spices and a sprinkle of salt and pepper.
2. Prepare by having the bowl of beaten egg ready, and the macadamia/spice mix spread out on a plate.
3. Lightly coat each chicken nibble in the beaten egg.
4. Transfer straight to the plate of macadamia nuts and thoroughly coat.
5. Drizzle some olive oil into the Crock Pot.
6. Lay the chicken nibbles in a single layer (if possible) into the Crock Pot.
7. Set the temperature to HIGH.
8. Cook for 2 hours, turning once, after the 1 hour mark.
9. Heat some olive oil in a fry pan or skillet.
10. Transfer the cooked chicken nibbles from the Crock Pot to the hot skillet, fry on both sides for 2 minutes a side until crispy and golden.
11. Serve on a platter with any dip of your choice, garlic aioli would be divine!.

Smoked fish dip

This dip is creamy, salty, and completely addictive. Serve with celery, capsicum, and carrot slices, (and some bread for your non-Keto guests!). Serve warm, with a sprinkling of fresh parsley on top.

Serves: makes 1 large bowl, about 6 – 8 people as a starter
Time: approximately 1 hour

Ingredients:
- 1 cup cream cheese
- 1 cup sour cream
- 2/3 cup smoked fish, (trout or salmon work wonders), flaked
- ½ cup grated cheddar cheese
- 2 garlic cloves, crushed
- 1 lemon
- Fresh parsley, finely chopped

Method:
1. Place cream cheese, sour cream, fish, garlic, zest and juice of 1 lemon in a medium-sized bowl, mix to combine.
2. Drizzle some oil into the Crock Pot.
3. Pour the smoked fish dip into the Crock Pot and spread to evenly cover the bottom of the pot.
4. Sprinkle the cheddar cheese over the dip.
5. Place the lid onto the pot and set the temperature to LOW.
6. Cook for 1 hour, the cheese on top should melt.
7. Remove the dip and serve in a bowl with a sprinkling of parsley over the top.
8. Serve warm with an assortment of fresh veggie sticks.

Warm cheese dip

Your guests will go crazy for this amazing dip! Or perhaps it's just for you and a loved on for a special occasion? Either way, this is an incredibly easy and delicious Keto-friendly dip. Serve with freshly sliced veggies for the Keto dieters, and some bread for the carb eaters!

Serves: makes one large bowl of dip, serves about 6 people
Time: approximately

Ingredients:
- 1 cup cream cheese, room temperature (take out of the fridge an hour before making the dip)
- 1 cup grated cheddar cheese
- 1 cup grated mozzarella
- 1 spring onion, finely chopped
- 2 garlic cloves, crushed
- 4 tbsp heavy cream
- 1 tsp chili powder (optional)

Method:
1. In the Crock Pot, mix together the cream cheese, cheddar, mozzarella, spring onion, garlic, chili, and cream.
2. Place the lid onto the pot and set the temperature at LOW.
3. Cook the dip for 4 hours – after 1 hour, give the dip a good stir to combine, as the cheese will have melted by then.
4. After the 4 hours, remove the Pot from the Crock Pot unit and serve as is. Otherwise, spoon the dip out of the pot and place into a serving bowl.
5. Serve with fresh veggies such as carrots, capsicum, radish, cucumber, and celery.

Lettuce boats with beef mince, parmesan, and pumpkin seeds

Cos lettuce is the perfect edible serving dish for appetizers and starters! These lettuce "boats" are filled with gorgeous beef mince, salty parmesan, and crunchy pumpkin seeds. If you don't have coz lettuce, use any other lettuce you can find, as long as it's sturdy enough and small enough for a small party snack.

Serves: 6 as a starter
Time: approximately 4 hours

Ingredients:
- 12 cos lettuce leaves (the outer and middle leaves are best, about 2 cos lettuces will suffice)
- 1 lb beef mince
- 2 garlic cloves, crushed
- ½ cup grated parmesan cheese
- ¼ cup pumpkin seeds

Method:
1. Drizzle some olive oil into the Crock Pot.
2. Add the beef mince, garlic, parmesan, salt, and pepper and stir to combine.
3. Add the lid to the pot and set the temperature to HIGH.
4. Cook for 2 hours or until the beef has cooked through and the parmesan has melted.
5. Fill each lettuce cup with a large spoonful of warm mince mixture and sprinkle the pumpkin seeds over the top.
6. Serve on a platter with a drizzle of olive oil and a sprinkling of sea salt and freshly cracked pepper.

Red pepper dip with warming spices and avocado oil

Yes, another dip recipe! Dips are just so easy to make in the Crock Pot, and even easier to serve. This dip uses the sweet deliciousness of red peppers, and the warming sensation of spices. Of course, you can replace the avocado oil with olive oil or coconut oil!

Serves: makes one large bowl of dip, about 6 – 8 servings
Time: approximately 2 hours

Ingredients:
- 6 red peppers (capsicums), seeds and core removed, cut into small chunks
- 3 garlic cloves, crushed
- 1 tsp dried chili flakes
- 1 tsp paprika
- ½ tsp cumin
- ½ tsp dried coriander
- 1 lemon
- ¾ cup sour cream

Method:
1. Drizzle some avocado oil into the Crock Pot.
2. Add the peppers, garlic, all of the spices, salt, pepper, and the finely grated zest of half a lemon to the pot, then add 2 tablespoons of water, stir to combine.
3. Add the lid to the pot and set the temperature to HIGH.
4. Cook for 3 hours or until the capsicum is very soft.
5. Leave to cool slightly.
6. With a hand-held stick blender, blend the peppers until a smooth dip forms.
7. Stir the sour cream and juice of half a lemon into the pepper dip.
8. Serve with a sprinkle of finely chopped fresh parsley and a drizzle of avocado oil.

Sushi-inspired cucumber, avocado, and chicken rolls

These roles are inspired by sushi, as they are rolled in seaweed, but without the rice. I love using toasted sesame seeds with these rolls as they give a lovely, nutty flavor. Serve with soy sauce and wasabi!

Serves: 8 as a starter
Time: approximately 4 and a half hours

Ingredients:
- 3 large chicken breasts, cut into 8 pieces each
- 2 tbsp soy sauce
- 1 tsp sesame oil
- 2 tbsp toasted sesame seeds
- 3 nori sheets
- 1 large avocado, cut into slices
- ½ cucumber, cut into slices
- 3 tbsp Japanese mayonnaise (optional)

Method:
1. Drizzle some olive oil into the Crock Pot.
2. Add the chicken pieces to the pot and sprinkle with salt and pepper.
3. Pour the soy sauce, sesame oil, and sesame seeds over the chicken and stir until the chicken is coated.
4. Place the lid onto the pot and set the temperature to LOW.
5. Cook for 4 hours.
6. Prepare to make the rolls by having the sliced avocado and cucumber ready, and the nori sheets laid on a sushi mat or chopping board.
7. Place a row of cooked chicken pieces on to the nori sheet, on the bottom third of the sheet, then place a row of avocado and cucumber on top of the chicken.
8. If using Japanese mayonnaise, place a thin line of it on top of the ingredients now.
9. Sprinkle some extra sesame seeds onto the filling.
10. Carefully roll the nori with the filling tightly inside.
11. Seal the edge with some water and your finger tip.
12. Slice each roll into 8 pieces.
13. Serve on a platter with a side of soy sauce and wasabi!

Mini pumpkin soups

I think mini cups of creamy pumpkin soup are a great way to start a meal or dinner party. A small amount of pumpkin is perfectly fine on the Keto diet, so go ahead and enjoy one of these warm and satisfying starters.

Serves: 8 as a starter
Time: approximately 4 hours

Ingredients:
- 2 lb butternut pumpkin, peeled and chopped into chunks
- 1 onion, finely chopped
- 4 garlic cloves, crushed
- 2 cup chicken stock
- 2/3 cup heavy cream

Method:
1. Drizzle some olive oil into the Crock Pot.
2. Add the pumpkin, onion, garlic, stock, salt, and pepper to the pot and stir to combine.
3. Place the lid onto the pot and set the temperature to HIGH.
4. Cook for 3 hours or until the pumpkin is completely soft.
5. Leave to cool slightly.
6. With a hand-held stick blender, whiz the soup until totally smooth.
7. Stir the cream through the soup and add salt and pepper to taste.
8. If you prefer a thinner soup, add more cream.
9. Serve in small serving cups or mugs with an extra dash of cream on top.

Spiced nut "snackers"

If you are hosting a game night, movie night, or any kind of event, these spiced nuts will be gone in a flash! The crunchy texture, spicy flavor, and utter "moreishness" will have you craving more and more. Use your favorite nuts! For Keto dieters, a few of these nuts will not harm your Ketosis whatsoever, in fact, the hit of fat will do you good!

Serves: makes 2 large jars of spiced nuts
Time: approximately 4 hours

Ingredients:

- 4 cups mixed nuts, the best Keto-friendly nuts are almonds, pecans, and macadamia nuts
- 2 tbsp butter, melted
- 2 tbsp coconut oil, melted
- 2 tsp cinnamon
- ½ tsp ground nutmeg
- 1 tsp sea salt
- Small pinch of curry powder

Method:

1. Place the butter, coconut oil, cinnamon, nutmeg, sea salt, and curry powder into the Crock Pot and stir to combine.
2. Add the nuts to the pot and stir until the nuts are coated.
3. Place the lid onto the Crock Pot and set the temperature to LOW.
4. Cook for 3 hours.
5. If you prefer crispier nuts, toss the cooked nuts in a hot skillet with the remaining liquid from the Crock Pot before serving in small bowls, otherwise, remove from the Crock Pot and place in bowls.
6. Serve once slightly cooled.

Chicken and cabbage "dumplings"

These are basically dumplings without the pastry casing. Well actually...they're more like meat balls, but I like to pretend they are dumplings! I always serve these with two dipping sauces: garlic mayonnaise, and chili vinegar. You can skip the final step and serve them straight from the Crock Pot without sautéing them first.

Serves: 6 as a starter
Time: approximately 2 hours

Ingredients:
- 1 lb minced chicken
- 2 cups shredded cabbage
- 2 garlic cloves, crushed
- 1 spring onion, finely chopped
- 1 egg, lightly beaten
- 1 tsp sesame oil
- 2 tbsp soy sauce

Method:
1. In a large bowl, add the minced chicken, cabbage, garlic, spring onion, egg, sesame oil and soy sauce, mix to thoroughly combine.
2. Roll the mixture into about 18 even-sized balls.
3. Drizzle some olive oil into the Crock Pot.
4. Lay the dumplings into the pot in one even layer if possible.
5. Place the lid onto the pot and set the temperature to LOW.
6. Cook for 4 hours.
7. If you like crispier dumplings, heat some oil in a frying pan or skillet and fry the dumplings until the outside is golden and crispy.
8. Serve the dumplings on a platter, with some tooth picks and a range of sauces.

Mini lamb burgers

These mini burgers are ideal for parties. They are easy to eat with one hand, and are absolutely delicious. The lettuce "buns" hold together the ingredients brilliantly, and keep you well within your Keto boundaries.

Serves: makes 12 mini burgers
Time: approximately 3 hours

Ingredients:
- 1 lb minced lamb
- 3 garlic cloves, crushed
- 1 tsp mixed dried herbs
- 1 egg, lightly beaten
- 12 small slices/pieces of cheddar cheese
- 12 small lettuce leaves (cos would be fine)
- ½ cup mayonnaise
- 12 cucumber slices

Method:
1. In a medium-sized bowl, mix together the minced lamb, garlic, dried herbs, egg, salt, and pepper until combined.
2. Roll the mixture into 12 balls, and flatted with your palms to create a mini patty.
3. Drizzle some olive oil into the Crock Pot.
4. Place the lamb patties into the pot.
5. Place a slice of cheese on top of each patty.
6. Place the lid onto the pot and set the temperature to HIGH.
7. Cook for 3 hours.
8. Preheat the oven to 200 degrees Celsius (392 Fahrenheit), on the GRILL setting.
9. Place the cheese-covered patties onto an oven tray and place into the hot oven.
10. Grill for a few minutes until the cheese is bubbling and the edges of the patties are golden.
11. Assemble the burgers by placing a patty onto a lettuce leave, then placing a dollop of mayonnaise on top, followed by a cucumber slice, fold the lettuce over so that it encases the fillings.
12. Serve on a platter!

Breakfast

These Keto-friendly breakfast recipes are packed with veggies and healthy fats. If you're a reluctant breakfast eater, hopefully these recipes will inspire you to start eating a decent morning meal!

Bacon and spiced egg bake

Bacon and eggs, yes, it's a classic! This recipe adds a touch of spice to the eggs to give it something special. Use free range eggs and responsibly-farmed bacon!

Serves: 2
Time: approximately 1 hour

Ingredients:
- 4 eggs
- 4 slices streaky bacon
- ½ tsp mixed spices – paprika, chili powder, cumin
- Fresh parsley, finely chopped

Method:
1. Drizzle some olive oil into the Crock pot.
2. In a small bowl, lightly beat the eggs.
3. Add the spices to the eggs with a pinch of salt and pepper, stir to combine.
4. Lay the bacon slices on the bottom of the Crock Pot.
5. Pour the egg mixture over the bacon.
6. Place the lid onto the pot and set the temperature to LOW.
7. Cook for 1 hour or until the egg has set.
8. Heat some oil in a skillet or frying pan.
9. Transfer the bacon and eggs in one piece to the pan and fry for 2 minutes until the bacon is crispy.
10. Serve on 2 plates with a sprinkling of fresh parsley.

Ricotta cheese and almond mini pancakes

Ricotta cheese gives such a light and fluffy texture to these mini pancakes. The ground almonds give a lovely nuttiness and are full of healthy fats. Serve with a few berries and some lemon juice...what a gorgeous breakfast!

Serves: 2
Time: approximately 2 hours

Ingredients:
- 1 cup ricotta cheese
- 2 eggs
- ½ cup ground almonds
- 1 tsp vanilla extract
- 1 tsp cinnamon

Method:
1. In a medium-sized bowl, mix together the ricotta cheese, eggs, ground almonds, vanilla, cinnamon, and a small pinch of salt.
2. Drizzle some coconut oil into the Crock Pot.
3. Place dollops of pancake batter into the pot, don't worry if the pancakes run together a bit, you can simply detach them when you flip them.
4. Place the lid onto the pot and set the temperature to LOW.
5. Cook for 2 hours, flip the pancakes once, after the 1-hour mark.
6. Serve the pancakes warm, with a few fresh berries!.

Cheesy green omelet

This omelet gets its "green" name from the glorious baby spinach folded throughout. Eggs and leafy greens are a perfect way to start a Keto-friendly day. The cheese makes this omelet a bit decadent and gooey! Throw this in the Crock Pot when you get up, and leave it while you get ready.

Serves: 2
Time: approximately 1 hour

Ingredients:
- 4 eggs
- 2 cups fresh spinach, chopped
- ½ cup grated cheddar

Method:
1. Rinse the spinach and place it in a microwave-proof bow, cover the bowl and place in the microwave on high for 1 minute, or until wilted.
2. Squeeze the moisture out of the spinach and finely chop.
3. In a medium-sized bowl, lightly beat the eggs, add the spinach, cheese, salt and pepper, stir to combine.
4. Drizzle some olive oil into the Crock Pot.
5. Pour the egg/spinach mixture into the pot.
6. Place the lid onto the pot and set the temperature to LOW.
7. Cook for about 1 hour or until the egg has set to your liking.
8. Serve with a side of bacon and a sprinkle of fresh herbs!

Salmon and asparagus with herb butter

Salmon and asparagus make such an elegant pair. The asparagus are cooked slowly, with a sprinkling of garlic and chili to really make the flavor pop. The herb butter melts over the hot asparagus, forming a buttery sauce. I used smoked salmon, and simply place it on top of the asparagus before serving.

Serves: 4
Time: approximately 2 hours

Ingredients:
- 20 asparagus spears, (5 spears per person)
- 2 garlic cloves, crushed
- 1 tsp dried chili flakes
- 3 tbsp butter
- 2 tsp fresh herbs, finely chopped – use any herbs you have, I like rosemary, mint, oregano, thyme and sage
- 3 ounces smoked salmon

Method:
1. Drizzle some olive oil into the Crock Pot.
2. Lay the asparagus into the Crock Pot and sprinkle the garlic, chili, salt, and pepper over the top, toss the asparagus to combine.
3. Drizzle some more olive oil over the asparagus.
4. Place the lid onto the pot and set the temperature to HIGH.
5. Cook for 2 hours.
6. While the asparagus cooks, prepare the herb butter by mixing the butter, herbs, salt, and pepper together and store in the fridge until needed.
7. Once the asparagus has finished cooking, place on plates while hot, with a dollop of herb butter on top.
8. Drape the smoked salmon over the asparagus and serve immediately.

Zucchini, mushroom, and avocado stack

I love that "stack" is now a common way to describe a breakfast dish! It perfectly describes this dish, as it's a gorgeous stack of Keto-friendly ingredients. You can add any other ingredients you like; haloumi or bacon would be divine.

Serves: 4
Time: approximately 2 hours

Ingredients:
- 2 large zucchinis, cut into 4 slices each (lengthways)
- 4 large Portobello mushrooms
- 2 garlic cloves, crushed
- 1 tbsp butter
- 1 large avocado, cut into slices

Method:
1. Drizzle some olive oil into the Crock Pot.
2. Lay the zucchini slices and mushrooms into the pot and sprinkle the garlic over the vegetables.
3. Sprinkle some salt, pepper, and extra olive oil over the vegetables.
4. Place a small knob of butter on top of each mushroom.
5. Place the lid onto the pot and set the temperature to HIGH.
6. Cook for about 1.5 hours.
7. Once the vegetables are cooked, layer them on 4 plates in a "tower", stack the towers by alternating zucchini, mushroom, and avocado slices.
8. Sprinkle with fresh herbs if you wish.
9. Serve warm.

Toasted nut, seed, and cinnamon sprinkles

This crunchy concoction is great for sprinkling over yoghurt and berries, or simply for nibbling on when you fancy a tiny snack! You can add any other nuts or seeds you like.

Serves: makes 1 large jar of sprinkles
Time: approximately 2 hours

Ingredients:
- 2 cups mixed nuts – almonds, macadamias, and pecans are best for Keto dieters
- 1 cup mixed seeds – pumpkin seeds, sesame seeds, sunflower seeds, chia seeds
- 3 tbsp coconut oil, melted
- 1 tsp sea salt
- 1 tsp cinnamon

Method:
1. In a large bowl, add the nuts, seeds, coconut oil, sea salt, and cinnamon, stir to combine, the nuts and seeds should be coated with oil and cinnamon.
2. Tip the nut/seed mixture into the crock pot and set the temperature to HIGH.
3. Cook for 2 hours, stirring every half hour.
4. If you prefer crispier nuts, you can finish them off by sautéing them in a frying pan over a high heat for about 1 minute, otherwise, simply leave them on a tray to cool before storing in a large jar.
5. Sprinkle over yoghurt, or eat as a quick snack!

Ricotta, spinach, and sausage cakes

Ricotta makes another appearance in the breakfast section! Spinach and sausage join the ricotta to make a truly delicious breakfast "cake". Serve with thick Greek yoghurt on the side, drizzled with olive oil. Use good quality sausages with no added carbs. Chorizo would also work really well!

Serves: 4
Time: approximately 2 hours

Ingredients:
- 1 ½ cups ricotta cheese
- 1 cup baby spinach, finely chopped
- 2 sausages, cut into small pieces
- 2 eggs

Method:
1. Heat some olive oil in a small skillet or pan, sauté the sausage pieces until golden.
2. In a medium-sized bowl, add the ricotta cheese, spinach, sausage pieces, egg, salt, and pepper, mix to combine.
3. Drizzle some olive oil into the Crock Pot.
4. Shape the ricotta mixture into 8 "cakes" (like a patty).
5. Place the cakes into the Crock Pot.
6. Place the lid onto the pot and set the temperature to HIGH.
7. Cook for 2 hours, turning once, after the 1-hour mark.
8. Serve while hot, with any sides you like. A side of grilled tomatoes and avocado would make for a super sophisticated breakfast!

Stuffed breakfast peppers

These stuffed peppers not only taste amazing, but they look elegant too! This is a great recipe to use when you feel like getting some extra veggies, but also want something tasty and satisfying.

Serves: 4
Time: approximately 2 hours

Ingredients:
- 4 large red peppers
- 3 eggs, lightly beaten
- 3 ounces feta cheese, cut into small chunks
- 2 cups baby spinach, roughly chopped
- 2 slices streaky bacon, chopped into small pieces

Method:
1. In a small bowl, mix together the eggs, feta cheese, spinach, bacon pieces, salt, and pepper.
2. Prepare the peppers by cutting around the stalk and removing it, reach into the peppers and remove the seeds.
3. Carefully pour the egg mixture evenly into each pepper, (don't worry if they're only half filled).
4. Drizzle some olive oil into the Crock Pot
5. Place the filled peppers carefully into the pot, prop them up against each other so they stay upright while cooking.
6. Place the lid onto the pot and set the temperature to HIGH.
7. Cook for 2 hours.
8. Remove the filled peppers from the Crock Pot and serve while hot.

Berry cheat treats

While these are called "treats", they are completely Keto-friendly! Keep these in the fridge to grab when you feel like something a bit sweet and naughty for breakfast or morning tea.

Serves: about 9 (makes 18 treats)
Time: approximately 2 hours

Ingredients:
- 2 cups fresh berries – (strawberries, raspberries, and blueberries are great), chopped
- ½ lb cream cheese
- 1 egg, lightly beaten
- ¾ cup chopped almonds
- ½ tsp cinnamon
- 1 tsp coconut oil, melted

Method:
1. Add the berries, cream cheese, egg, and cinnamon to a medium-sized bowl and stir to combine.
2. Have the chopped almonds ready by spreading them onto a place.
3. Roll the berry mixture into 18 balls.
4. Roll each ball in the chopped almonds until coated.
5. Rub the bottom of the Crock Pot with the melted coconut oil.
6. Place the berry balls into the crock pot in a single layer.
7. Place the lid onto the pot and set the temperature at LOW.
8. Cook for 2 hours, turning the balls once, after the first hour.
9. Once cooked, leave to cool on a rack before storing in an airtight container in the fridge.
10. Eat when you need a super-quick breakfast treat!

Warm ricotta, cream, berry and macadamia whip

This recipe is like a mash-up of my favorite things...cream, berries, macadamia nuts, and ricotta cheese. It could be enjoyed as a dessert, but I like it for breakfast! It's amazing with a sprinkling of toasted nut sprinkles.

Serves: 6
Time: approximately 2 hours

Ingredients:
- 2 cups ricotta cheese
- 1 cup fresh berries, chopped (strawberries and raspberries are wonderful)
- ½ cup toasted macadamia nuts, chopped
- 1 tsp cinnamon
- 1 tsp coconut oil, melted
- 1 cup cream, lightly whipped

Method:
1. In a medium-sized bowl, mix together the ricotta cheese, berries, cinnamon, and macadamia nuts.
2. Rub the bottom of the Crock Pot with the melted coconut oil.
3. Pour the ricotta mixture into the Crock Pot.
4. Place the lid onto the pot and set the temperature at LOW.
5. Cook for 2 hours.
6. Remove the mixture from the pot and place into a bowl, leave to cool.
7. Add the whipped cream and fold through, with a few more fresh berries.
8. Store in the fridge, covered.

Haloumi, chorizo and Brussel's sprout breakfast bowl

Any dish that can be thrown in a bowl and served with a fork and a sprinkling of pepper has my tick of approval! This breakfast bowl is salty, cheesy, and wholesome.

Serves: 4
Time: approximately 4 hours

Ingredients:
- ½ lb haloumi cheese, cut into small pieces
- 2 chorizo sausages, cut into small pieces
- 16 Brussel's sprouts, cut in half
- 2 garlic cloves, crushed
- 4 eggs

Method:
1. Drizzle some olive oil into the Crock Pot.
2. Add the haloumi, chorizo, Brussel's sprouts, garlic, salt, and pepper to the Crock Pot, stir to combine.
3. Place the lid onto the pot and set the temperature at HIGH.
4. Cook for 2 hours or until the sprouts are cooked.
5. If you wish, you can finish the dish off by quickly sautéing the whole lot in a hot fry pan or skillet until golden and crispy.
6. Serve on 4 plates, with a poached egg on top.
7. Serve while hot!

Mushroom and brie "melters"

These little morsels look so lovely on a platter, with a dash of fresh herbs for color. Despite being unbelievably easy to make, they are super tasty and impressive. You don't need to splash out on expensive brie, the good ole supermarket stuff does the trick!

Serves: 6 as a starter
Time: approximately 2 hours

Ingredients:
- 12 medium-sized brown mushrooms (Swiss Browns are ideal)
- 1/3 lb wheel of brie, cut or torn into 12 pieces
- 3 garlic cloves, crushed
- 2 tsp chopped fresh or dried parsley

Method:
1. Drizzle some olive oil into the Crock Pot.
2. Lay the mushrooms on a board and rub them with olive oil.
3. Sprinkle the crushed garlic, herbs, salt, and pepper evenly over the mushrooms.
4. Place a piece of brie on top of each mushroom.
5. Very carefully transfer the mushrooms to the Crock Pot and lay in a single layer.
6. Place the lid onto the pot and set the temperature to HIGH.
7. Cook for 2 hours.
8. Heat a small drizzle of olive oil on a fry pan or skillet.
9. Transfer the cooked mushrooms to the skillet and sauté for about 1 minute to get the mushrooms golden on the bottom (you can skip this step if you prefer softer mushrooms, but I like the slightly charred flavor) .
10. Serve on a platter with a sprinkling of grated parmesan cheese if you want to get extra fancy!

Chocolate and hazelnut pancakes

I had you at "chocolate", right? These pancakes are so nutritious and Keto-friendly, but they taste like a glorious breakfast/dessert hybrid! I like to serve them with whipped cream and fresh berries for an all-out decadent breakfast or brunch.

Serves: 4
Time: approximately 1 hour

Ingredients:
- 1 cup ricotta cheese
- 2 eggs
- ½ cup ground hazelnuts
- ¼ cup unsweetened cocoa powder
- ½ tsp baking powder
- 1 tsp cinnamon
- ½ cup blueberries (fresh or frozen)

Method:
1. In a medium-sized bowl, mix together the ricotta cheese, eggs, ground hazelnuts, cocoa powder, cinnamon, and a pinch of salt, don't over mix.
2. Fold through the blue berries.
3. Drizzle some coconut oil into the Crock Pot.
4. Drop small dollops of mixture into the pot, don't worry if it all runs together, you can separate the pancakes when you flip them.
5. Place the lid onto the pot and set the temperature to HIGH.
6. Cook for an hour, turning once, after the half hour mark.
7. The pancakes might not look perfect or pretty, as they can sometimes run together, but they will taste divine!
8. Serve with yoghurt or cream, and fresh berries.

Cauliflower breakfast cake with capsicum and chorizo

This is a big, rustic, delicious cake of breakfast goodness! Serve it in rough chunks, with a poached egg on top. You'll never need to go to a café again...because this is just as good, if not better!

Serves: 6
Time: approximately 4 hours

Ingredients:
- ½ head of cauliflower, roughly chopped
- 3 garlic cloves, crushed
- 2 red capsicums, seeds and core removed, roughly chopped
- 2 zucchinis, sliced
- 2 chorizo sausages, cut into chunks
- ½ cup grated cheddar cheese
- Fresh parsley, finely chopped

Method:
1. Drizzle the Crock Pot with olive oil.
2. Add the garlic, cauliflower, capsicums, zucchinis, and chorizo to the pot, sprinkle with salt and pepper.
3. Drizzle some more olive oil over the vegetables, then sprinkle the grated cheese over the top.
4. Place the lid onto the pot and set the temperature to LOW.
5. Cook for 4 hours.
6. If you like, you can transfer the whole dish from the Crock Pot to a hot skillet or fry pan to finish off once it has cooked in the Crock Pot, this will ensure a crispy, golden finish.
7. Serve on a plate with a poached egg, and a healthy sprinkling of fresh parsley.

Keto "big breakfast" starring avocado, feta, and bacon

This is the breakfast to choose when you're feeling a little under the weather, perhaps you over-indulged on your low-carb beverages the night before? Creamy avocado, salty feta, and irresistible bacon will surely satisfy your cravings!

Serves: 4
Time: approximately 2 hours

Ingredients:
- 5 eggs, lightly beaten
- 8 slices of streaky bacon
- 1 red capsicum, seeds and core removed, sliced
- 5 ounces feta cheese, crumbled or chopped into small pieces
- 2 avocadoes, sliced
- 1 lemon

Method:
1. Drizzle some olive oil into the Crock Pot.
2. Pour the egg into the pot and place the capsicum, feta, bacon, salt, and pepper on top of the egg.
3. Place the lid on the pot and set the temperature to LOW.
4. Cook for 2 hours.
5. Once cooked, cut into 4 pieces, (like a pizza or quiche) and place on 4 plates.
6. Place the avocado slices on top, and drizzle with some olive oil and a squeeze of lemon juice for tartness.
7. Serve immediately!

Soups & Stews

Soups, stews, and the Crock Pot go together like peas and carrots. Throw the ingredients into the pot, set the temperature, and leave it to work wonders! Return from work or leisure to find a delicious, hot soup or stew to enjoy.

Chicken, chili, and lime soupy-stew

I called this a soupy-stew because it's 50/50 between a soup and a stew. The chili, lime, and coriander give a lovely Mexican flavor to the tender chicken, and tomato base.

Serves: 6
Time: approximately 6 hours

Ingredients:
- 6 chicken thighs, skin on, boneless
- 3 garlic cloves, crushed
- 1 small onion, finely chopped
- 2 tins chopped tomatoes
- 1 red chili, finely chopped
- 1 chicken stock cube
- 2 limes
- Large handful of fresh coriander, chopped

Method:
1. Drizzle some olive oil into the Crock Pot.
2. Place the chicken, garlic, onion, tomatoes, chili, stock cube, juice of 2 limes, 1 cup water, and half the chopped coriander to the pot.
3. Sprinkle with salt and pepper.
4. Place the lid onto the pot and set the temperature to LOW.
5. Cook for 6 hours.
6. Once the soupy-stew has cooked, gently separate the chicken pieces with two forks to shred.
7. Serve while hot, with a couple of slices of avocado on top.

Creamy smoked salmon soup

A small serving of this soup is enough, as it's very rich and decadent. The healthy fats and oils in the salmon are great for skin and brain health, and the high fat content from the cream is ideal for Keto dieters.

Serves: 6
Time: approximately 3 hours

Ingredients:
- ½ lb smoked salmon, roughly chopped
- 4 garlic cloves, crushed
- 1 small onion, finely chopped
- 1 leek, finely chopped
- 2 cups heavy cream
- 1 fish stock cube

Method:
1. Drizzle some oil into the Crock Pot.
2. Add the onion, garlic, salmon, leek, stock cube, and 1 cup of water into the pot.
3. Place the lid onto the pot and set the temperature to LOW.
4. Cook for 2 hours.
5. Stir the cream through the soup and continue to cook for a further 1 hour.
6. Serve with a sprinkling of freshly cracked pepper, I don't add extra salt because the smoked salmon is salty enough for me.

Roasted sweet pepper soup

Capsicums are a wonderful soup ingredient, as they are gorgeously sweet when cooked. Delicate spices and garlic give a lovely zing of flavor to this vibrant soup.

Serves: 6
Time: approximately 4 hours

Ingredients:
- 6 red capsicums, core and seeds removed, roughly chopped
- 2 celery sticks, chopped into chunks
- 6 garlic cloves, finely chopped
- 1 onion, finely chopped
- 1 chicken stock cube
- 1 tsp cumin
- 1 tsp ground coriander
- ½ cup sour cream

Method:
1. Drizzle some olive oil into the Crock Pot.
2. Add the capsicum, celery, garlic, onion, stock cube, cumin, coriander, salt, pepper, and 2 cups of water to the pot.
3. Place the lid onto the pot and set the temperature to LOW.
4. Cook for 6 hours.
5. With a hand-held stick blender, blend the soup until smooth.
6. Stir the sour cream through the soup before serving.
7. Serve while hot.

Lamb and rosemary stew

Soft lamb and woody rosemary in a rich stew gravy. Serve with buttered cauliflower rice. Leave in the pot all day while you are out and about, and come home to a delicious aroma and ready-to-go dinner.

Serves: 6
Time: approximately 8 hours

Ingredients:

- 2 lb boneless lamb, cut into cubes
- 1 onion, roughly chopped
- 4 garlic cloves, finely chopped
- 2 tsp dried rosemary
- 1 lamb stock cube

Method:

1. Drizzle some olive oil into the Crock Pot.
2. Brown the lamb in an oiled fry pan or skillet for about 2 minutes.
3. Add the lamb, onion, garlic, rosemary, stock cube, salt, pepper, and 3 cups of water to the pot.
4. Place the lid onto the pot and set the time to LOW.
5. Cook for 8 hours.
6. Remove the lid, stir, and serve while hot.

Beef and onion stew

Beef and onion stew can't be beat. Affordable, tasty, nourishing, and low carb, this is a great recipe to have up your sleeve for any occasion. Stewing beef is cheap and great for slow cooking.

Serves: 6
Time: approximately 10 hours

Ingredients:
- 2 lb boneless stewing beef, cut into cubes
- 2 onions, roughly chopped
- 5 garlic cloves, crushed
- 1 beef stock cube
- 1 tsp dried mixed herbs

Method:
1. Drizzle the Crock Pot with olive oil.
2. Brown the beef in an oiled fry pan or skillet for about 2 minutes to seal.
3. Place the beef, onions, garlic, stock cube, salt, pepper, herbs, and 3 cups of water to the pot.
4. Place the lid onto the pot.
5. Set the temperature to LOW.
6. Cook for 10 hours.
7. Remove the lid, stir the stew, and serve while hot, with a side of greens and mashed cauliflower.

Stewed pork

Stewed pork can be eaten as a main dish, with a simple side of veggies, or it can be used as the basis of other dishes such as burgers and sandwiches, (Keto-friendly ones, of course!). I like to serve this pork with a dollop of thick Greek yoghurt and a pile of greens.

Serves: 6
Time: approximately 8 hours

Ingredients:
- 2 lb pork loin, cut into cubes
- 1 onion, finely chopped
- 4 garlic cloves, crushed
- 3 cups chicken stock
- 1 tsp dried spices – cumin, coriander, chili, turmeric

Method:
1. Drizzle some olive oil into the Crock Pot.
2. Add the pork, onion, garlic, stock, spices, salt, and pepper to the pot and stir to combine.
3. Place the lid onto the pot and set the temperature to LOW.
4. Cook for 8 hours.
5. Remove the lid, stir, and slightly break the pork apart with 2 forks for a smaller texture.
6. Serve hot with your favorite low-carb veggies!

Coconut, white fish, and fresh coriander soup

You could call this a curry...but I like to think of it as a soup, as it's served without rice or noodles, (do you follow my logic?). Use any fresh white fish you can find locally, I use snapper. You could also use fresh salmon fillets for this dish, but I think it's lovely and light with white fish.

Serves: 6
Time: approximately 3 hours

Ingredients:
- 2 lb white fish, cut into chunks
- 4 garlic cloves, crushed
- 1 onion, finely chopped
- 2 tsp fresh ginger, finely grated
- 2 tbsp curry paste (green or red, choose a high-quality paste)
- 3 cups full-fat coconut milk
- 1 lime
- Large handful of fresh coriander, roughly chopped

Method:
1. Drizzle some olive oil into the Crock Pot.
2. Add the fish, garlic, onion, ginger, curry paste, coconut milk, juice of one lime, and half of the coriander to the pot, stir to combine.
3. Place the lid on the pot and set the temperature to LOW.
4. Cook for 5 hours.
5. Remove the lid, stir, and dish into bowls.
6. Sprinkle with the remaining fresh coriander!

Bacon, paprika, and cauliflower soup

I just had to include a cauliflower soup in this section, because it truly is one of my all-time favorite soups. The bacon adds a delicious...bacon-ness! (You know what I mean), and the paprika is smoky and sweet in the best way.

Serves: 6
Time: approximately 4 hours

Ingredients:
- 1 large head of cauliflower, cut into chunks
- 4 garlic cloves, crushed
- 1 onion, finely chopped
- 5 slices streaky bacon, cut into small pieces
- 2 cups chicken stock
- 1 tsp smoked paprika
- 1 tsp chili powder (optional)
- 1 cup heavy cream

Method:
1. Drizzle some olive oil into the pot.
2. Add the cauliflower, garlic, onion, bacon, stock, paprika, chili, salt, and pepper to the pot, stir to combine.
3. Place the lid onto the pot and set the temperature to HIGH.
4. Cook for 4 hours.
5. With a hand-held stick blender, blend until smooth.
6. Mix the cream into the soup.
7. Serve while hot, with a sprinkling of paprika on top!

Cheesy broccoli and leek soup

I find something so decadent and almost naughty about eating cheese in a soup, it's just so gooey and luxurious! This soup is full of nutrient-dense greens, and tastes incredible.

Serves: 6
Time: approximately 3 hours

Ingredients:
- 1 large head of broccoli, cut into small pieces
- 1 large leek, sliced
- 4 garlic cloves, finely chopped
- 2 cups vegetable or chicken stock
- 1 cup grated cheddar cheese
- 1 cup full-fat cream

Method:
1. Drizzle some olive oil into the Crock Pot.
2. Add the broccoli, leek, garlic, stock, salt, and pepper to the pot, stir to combine.
3. Place the lid onto the pot and set the temperature to HIGH.
4. Cook for 3 hours.
5. With a hand-held stick blender, blend the soup until smooth.
6. Add the cheese and cream to the soup and stir.
7. Place the lid back onto the pot and cook on HIGH for another hour, or until the cheese has melted.
8. Serve while hot!

Pumpkin and parmesan soup

This is a twist on that old classic, pumpkin soup. Parmesan cheese is so sharp and salty, it really lifts the sweet, velvety pumpkin.

Serves: 6
Time: approximately 4 hours

Ingredients:
- 1 butternut pumpkin, peeled and cubed
- 1 onion, finely chopped
- 4 garlic cloves, finely chopped
- 2 cups chicken stock
- ¾ cup grated parmesan cheese
- ½ cup heavy cream

Method:
1. Drizzle some olive oil into the Crock Pot.
2. Add the pumpkin, onion, garlic, stock, salt, and pepper to the pot, stir to combine.
3. Place the lid onto the pot and set the temperature to HIGH.
4. Cook for 4 hours.
5. With a hand-held stick blender, blend until smooth.
6. Stir the parmesan and cream into the hot soup and leave in the pot with the lid on for about twenty minutes, or until the cheese melts.
7. Serve while hot, with an extra grating of parmesan on top!

Chicken and egg soup

The "egg" part of this soup is added at the very end, and must be eaten straight away, so the yolk stays glorious and runny! The base of this soup is a gingery, spicy broth, with pieces of tender chicken.

Serves: 6
Time: approximately 4 hours

Ingredients:
- 4 chicken thighs, boneless, skinless, cut into medium-sized pieces
- 4 garlic cloves, finely chopped
- 1 red chili, finely chopped
- 1 tbsp finely grated fresh ginger
- 1 lemon
- 4 cups chicken stock
- 6 eggs (1 egg per person)
- Fresh coriander

Method:
1. Drizzle some olive oil into the Crock Pot.
2. Add the chicken, garlic, chili, ginger, juice of one lemon, stock, salt, and pepper to the pot, stir to combine.
3. Place the lid onto the pot and set the temperature to HIGH.
4. Cook for 4 hours.
5. Remove the lid and stir the soup.
6. At this stage, you can either crack the eggs straight into the hot soup to lightly poach, or you can simply poach them in water in a separate pot and place them into each serving bowl of soup.
7. Sprinkle each bowl of soup with fresh coriander!

Beef mince, tomato, and sausage chili

Since we cannot eat beans on Keto, I have treated us by making a chili with added MEAT! This chili is amazingly savory with the addition of sausages, chopped up and dispersed throughout. Choose good-quality, 100% meat sausages without additives and fillers.

Serves: 6 – 8
Time: approximately 8 hours

Ingredients:
- 2 lb minced beef
- 1 onion, finely chopped
- 4 garlic cloves, crushed
- 4 tomatoes, chopped
- 1 beef stock cube
- 1 tsp smoked paprika
- 1 tsp dried chili flakes (optional)
- 3 sausages, cut into pieces

Method:
1. Drizzle some olive oil into the Crock Pot.
2. Add the minced beef, onion, garlic, tinned tomatoes, stock cube, paprika, chili, sausages, salt, pepper, and one cup of water to the pot, stir to combine.
3. Place the lid onto the pot and set the temperature to LOW.
4. Cook for 8 hours.
5. Remove the lid, stir the chili, and serve while hot!

Chicken and spinach stew

Even if you're not so fond of spinach, you will love this stew. The spinach gives a lovely hit of color and a delicate freshness. The white wine and cream provide some sophisticated dimensions to this quick and easy dish.

Serves: 6 – 8
Time: approximately 8 hours

Ingredients:
- 2 lb chicken thighs and legs, bone in, skin on
- 2 cups spinach, roughly chopped
- 1 onion, finely chopped
- 6 garlic cloves, crushed
- 1 tsp dried tarragon
- 2 cups chicken stock
- ½ cup dry white wine
- ½ cup heavy cream

Method:
1. Drizzle some olive oil into the Crock Pot.
2. Add the chicken, spinach, onion, 4 cloves of garlic, stock, tarragon, salt, and pepper to the pot, stir to combine.
3. Add the lid to the pot and set the temperature to LOW.
4. Cook for 8 hours.
5. Drizzle some olive oil into a small pot and add the remaining 2 cloves of garlic.
6. Pour the wine into the pot and simmer until reduced.
7. Add the cream to the pot with the wine and stir to combine.
8. Remove the lid from the Crock Pot and stir the wine and cream mixture into the stew.
9. Serve while hot!

Layered "cheeseburger" stew

I call this "cheeseburger" stew because it tastes very reminiscent of a cheeseburger! I love burgers, but on Keto, we can't have the real deal...so why not enjoy the same flavors in a lovely bowl of stew? Give it a go and see what you think!

Serves: 6
Time: approximately 4 hours

Ingredients:
- 2 lb minced beef
- 1 onion, finely chopped
- 4 garlic cloves, crushed
- 1 beef stock cube
- 2 tomatoes, chopped
- ¼ cup sliced pickles or gherkins
- 2 cups grated cheddar cheese
- ½ head of iceberg lettuce, chopped
- 1 fresh tomato, sliced
- Mayonnaise – a dollop on the side of each serving
- Mustard – a dollop on the side of each serving

Method:
1. Drizzle some olive oil into the Crock Pot.
2. Add the minced beef, onion, garlic, stock cube, tinned tomatoes, salt, pepper, and 1 cup of water and stir to combine.
3. Place the lid onto the pot and set the temperature to HIGH.
4. Cook for 4 hours.
5. Remove the lid and stir, place a layer of pickles on top of the beef mince mixture.
6. Sprinkle the cheese over the pickle layer.
7. Place the lid back onto the pot and cook on HIGH for a further 30 minutes, or until the cheese has melted.
8. Serve with a side of shredded iceberg lettuce, freshly sliced tomato, and a dollop of mayonnaise and mustard.

Mozzarella, lamb, and eggplant stew

Eggplant and lamb make another star appearance, as I just can't get enough of the combination! This stew is rich, sweet, cheesy, and extremely satisfying. Serve with a side of greens and you will be a very happy eater indeed!

Serves: 6
Time: approximately 8 hours

Ingredients:
- 2 lb minced lamb
- 1 onion, finely chopped
- 4 garlic cloves, crushed
- 1 large eggplant, cut into small cubes
- 2 tomatoes, chopped
- 1 lamb stock cube
- 1 tsp dried rosemary
- 1 cup grated mozzarella

Method:
1. Drizzle some olive oil into the Crock Pot.
2. Add the minced lamb, onion, garlic, eggplant, stock cube, chopped tomatoes, rosemary, salt and pepper to the pot, stir to combine.
3. Place the lid onto the pot and set the temperature to HIGH.
4. Cook for 8 hours.
5. Remove the lid from the pot and stir the stew.
6. Sprinkle the mozzarella on top of the stew and place the lid back on the pot, cook for a further 30 minutes or until the cheese has melted.
7. Serve hot!

Kale and chicken broth soup

This soup is very light and hydrating, thanks to the nourishing chicken stock. I recommend this soup for when you or another Keto-dieter are feeling under the weather with a cold or flu. The Kale offers optimal nutrition, while the garlic, ginger, and chicken broth work to repair and nourish you back to health!

Serves: 4 – 6
Time: approximately 4 hours

Ingredients:
- 6 garlic cloves, finely chopped
- 3 tbsp grated fresh ginger
- 6 cups chicken stock
- 1 large chicken breast, cut into small strips
- 2 cups chopped fresh kale (stalks removed)

Method:
1. Drizzle some olive oil into the Crock Pot.
2. Add the garlic, ginger, stock, chicken breast, kale, salt, and pepper to the pot, stir to combine.
3. Place the lid onto the pot and set the temperature to HIGH.
4. Cook for 4 hours.
5. Serve this soup while steaming hot!.

Meat

The Crock Pot loves meat, and luckily enough...so does the Ketogenic diet. This recipe section contains chicken, beef, lamb, and pork. Make life easier by preparing a cut of meat and leaving it to slowly cook in the Crock Pot while you go about your day. All you need to do before serving is prepare some easy and healthy sides such as steamed veggies.

Slow cooker meat lover's pizza

Pizza doesn't need dough! In fact, my favorite parts of a pizza are the meat and cheese, which both get the Keto tick. This is great for an easy, fun Friday night meal.

Serves: 6
Time: approximately 4 hours

Ingredients:
- Half a head of cauliflower, blitzed in the food processor
- 1 egg, lightly beaten
- ½ cup grated parmesan cheese
- 18 slices of pepperoni or salami (or a mix of both)
- 1 green capsicum
- ½ cup passata or tomato puree
- 1 cup grated mozzarella cheese
- ½ cup grated cheddar cheese
- 1 tsp dried oregano

Method:
1. In a medium-sized bowl, mix the blitzed cauliflower, egg, parmesan, salt, and pepper until a thick "dough" forms.
2. Drizzle some olive oil into the Crock Pot.
3. Press the cauliflower mixture into the Crock Pot.
4. Spread the tomato passata or puree over the cauliflower base.
5. Sprinkle the mozzarella and cheddar over the tomato sauce.
6. Place the pepperoni and/or salami slices over the cheese.
7. Sprinkle the oregano over the meat slices.
8. Place the lid onto the pot and set the temperature at HIGH.
9. Cook for 4 hours, the cheese should be melted.
10. Serve as a "slice" with any sides you like!

Crock Pot beef shank

Beef shank is a wonderful cut of meat to use in the Crock Pot. Tender, fall-off-the-bone meat and delicious marrow melt together to form a rich and comforting dish.

Serves: 6
Time: approximately 8 hours

Ingredients:
- 2 lb beef shanks
- 1 onion, finely chopped
- 5 garlic cloves, finely chopped
- 2 cups red wine
- 3 cups beef stock
- Sprig of fresh rosemary

Method:
1. Heat some olive oil in a skillet or fry pan and brown the beef shanks until sealed on all sides.
2. Remove the beef shanks and set aside.
3. Pour the wine into the skillet and simmer to reduce.
4. Drizzle some olive oil into the Crock Pot.
5. Add the beef shanks, onion, garlic, reduced wine, stock, rosemary, salt, and pepper.
6. Secure the lid onto the pot and set the temperature to LOW.
7. Cook for 8 hours, the meat should be very tender.
8. Serve while hot, with a side of vegetables.

Stuffed chicken breasts

Chicken breasts are great and all, but I think they need a bit of help to become amazing. I think the best way to achieve that is to stuff them full of awesome things like cheese, olives, and spinach...yum!

Serves: 4 – 6
Time: approximately 4 hours

Ingredients:
- 4 large chicken breasts, skin off
- 4 garlic cloves, finely chopped
- ½ pound mozzarella cheese, sliced
- 12 black olives, pit removed, chopped into chunks
- 1 cup baby spinach, roughly chopped
- 2 tomatoes, chopped
- ½ tsp dried mixed herbs
- ½ cup grated mozzarella cheese

Method:
1. Slice the chicken breasts lengthways, so that a cavity opens (don't slice them into two pieces).
2. Rub the chicken breasts with olive oil and sprinkle with salt and pepper.
3. Stuff each breast with the garlic, mozzarella, olive, and spinach.
4. Place the chicken breasts into the Crock Pot and pour the tinned tomatoes over the top, sprinkle the mixed herbs over the top.
5. Set the temperature to HIGH.
6. Place the lid onto the pot and cook for 4 hours.
7. Sprinkle the extra mozzarella over the top and place the lid back onto the pot, cook until the cheese has melted.
8. Serve while hot!

Beef lasagna

If you have been craving lasagna but you assumed it was out of bounds on your Keto diet...think again! This lasagna uses gorgeous slices of veggies instead of pasta. The rich meat sauce and cheesy topping remains the same.

Serves: 6 – 8
Time: approximately 8 hours

Ingredients:
- 2 lb minced beef
- 1 onion, finely chopped
- 5 garlic cloves, finely chopped
- 2 tsp dried mixed herbs – oregano, rosemary, thyme
- 1 large eggplant, cut into slices width ways (rounds)
- 2 large zucchinis, cut into slices lengthways
- 2 cups baby spinach
- 4 tomatoes, chopped
- 2 cups grated cheddar cheese
- 1 cup grated mozzarella cheese
- 1 cup ricotta cheese

Method:
1. Heat some olive oil in a deep-sided frying pan.
2. Add the onions and garlic to the pan and sauté until soft.
3. Add the minced beef to the pan and cook for about 3 minutes to brown.
4. Add the tomatoes and mixed herbs to the beef and sprinkle with salt and pepper, cook for about 5 minutes.
5. Drizzle some olive oil into the Crock Pot.
6. Spread a layer of beef mixture into the pot.
7. Place a layer of eggplant over the beef.
8. Add another thin layer of beef mixture over the eggplant.
9. Place a layer of zucchini over the beef.
10. Add another layer of beef over the zucchini.
11. Place the spinach leaves over the beef.
12. Add the remaining beef mixture over the spinach.
13. In a large bowl, mix together the cheddar cheese, mozzarella, ricotta cheese, salt, and pepper.
14. Spread the cheese mixture over the lasagna.
15. Place the lid onto the pot and set the temperature to HIGH.
16. Cook for 4 hours.
17. Serve while hot!

Slow cooked savory mince

This dish my look and sound very simple, but it tastes completely delicious. The rich, gravy-like mince is lovely on its own on a cold Winter's night, or served over a pile over buttery cauliflower rice.

Serves: 6 – 8
Time: approximately 8 hours

Ingredients:
- 2 lb minced beef
- 1 large onion, finely chopped
- 4 garlic cloves, finely chopped
- 2 celery stalks, finely chopped
- 1 tbsp butter
- 3 cups beef stock

Method:
1. Heat some olive oil in a deep-sided frying pan.
2. Add the celery, onion and garlic to the pan and cook until soft.
3. Add the minced beef and cook for about 3 minutes to brown.
4. Drizzle some olive oil into the Crock Pot.
5. Add the mince mixture to the pot.
6. Add the butter, stock, salt, and pepper to the pot and stir to combine.
7. Place the lid onto the pot and set the temperature to LOW.
8. Cook for 8 hours.
9. Serve hot, with whatever accompaniments you like!

Lamb curry

Just like the name suggests, this is a simple, tasty, warming lamb curry. Slow cooking allows the lamb to become satisfyingly tender. This Keto-friendly curry freezes well, and leftovers can be enjoyed for lunch the next day! Madras curry paste works well, but use any kind you have on hand.

Serves: 6 – 8
Time: approximately 8 hours

Ingredients:
- 2 ½ lb boneless lamb (shoulder is a good cut to choose for this dish), cubed
- 2 onions, roughly chopped
- 5 garlic cloves, finely chopped
- 4 tbsp curry paste
- 1 lamb stock cube
- 2 ½ full-fat coconut milk
- 2 tomatoes, chopped
- Fresh coriander, roughly chopped
- Full-fat Greek yogurt, to serve

Method:
1. Heat some oil in skillet or pan.
2. Add the lamb to the hot pan and seal on all sides, about 3 minutes.
3. Drizzle some olive oil into the Crock Pot.
4. Add the lamb, onions, garlic, curry paste, salt, and pepper to the pot.
5. Stir to coat the lamb in curry paste.
6. Add the coconut milk, stock cube, chopped tomatoes, and 1 cup of water to the pot.
7. Place the lid onto the pot and set the temperature to LOW.
8. Cook for 8 hours.
9. Serve with a dollop of Greek yoghurt and fresh coriander.

Butter chicken

Another curry recipe! Crock Pot butter chicken is the best thing to come home to after a long day. Mild, creamy curry and juicy chunks of chicken...serve with cauliflower rice and fresh coriander (can you tell I love coriander yet?). Garam Masala is a mild Indian spice mix which can be found in most supermarkets.

Serves: 6 – 8
Time: approximately 8 hours

Ingredients:
- 2 lb boneless chicken thigh
- 6 garlic cloves, crushed
- 1 onion, finely chopped
- 2 tbsp grated fresh ginger
- Handful of fresh coriander, finely chopped
- 2 tbsp Garam Masala
- 2 tsp chili powder
- ½ cup full-fat Greek yoghurt
- 2 tbsp tomato paste
- 2 tomatoes, chopped
- 3 tbsp butter
- ½ cup heavy cream

Method:
1. In a large bowl, add the chicken thighs, garlic, onion, ginger, coriander, tomato paste, yoghurt, salt, and pepper. Stir to combine and thoroughly coat the chicken.
2. Leave the chicken to marinate for at least 4 hours, overnight is ideal.
3. Drizzle some olive oil into the Crock Pot.
4. Add the Garam Masala and chili powder to the pot and stir to create a paste.
5. Add the chicken and marinade to the pot and stir into the curry paste.
6. Add the tinned tomatoes, butter, salt, and pepper to the pot.
7. Place the lid onto the pot and set the temperature to LOW.
8. Cook for 8 hours.
9. Stir the cream into the curry before serving.
10. Serve with fresh coriander sprinkled on top.

Crock Pot whole chicken

A whole chicken is a glorious thing. Tear the meat off and use in sandwiches, salads, or simply eat cold with a lovely side salad. Get the bird cooking before you leave for work and come home to a pot of goodness!

Serves: makes 1 whole chicken
Time: approximately 6 hours

Ingredients:
- 1 medium-sized chicken
- 1 tsp fresh dried herbs
- 1 lemon
- 6 garlic cloves, skin kept on
- 2 onions, cut into rough chunks
- 3 celery sticks, cut into rough chunks
- ¾ cup chicken stock
- 3 tbsp butter

Method:
1. Drizzle some olive oil into the Crock Pot.
2. Prepare the chicken by rubbing with olive oil and sprinkling with dried herbs, salt, and pepper.
3. Stuff the lemon into the chicken cavity.
4. Add the onion chunks, celery chunks, and garlic cloves to the pot, pour the stock over the vegetables.
5. Lay the chicken on top of the vegetables.
6. Place a knob of butter on top of the chicken and press into the skin.
7. Place the lid onto the pot and set the temperature to HIGH.
8. Cook for 6 hours.
9. Remove the lid, take the chicken out of the pot and leave to rest on a board to cool slightly before serving!
10. Use the remaining liquid and vegetables from the pot to make a gravy by reducing in a pan and adding more liquid or thickeners if need be.

Pork pot roast

A juicy slice of slow cooked pork can't be beat. This is a super-simple recipe – minimal fuss, ultimate flavor. Serve however you like! A side of buttered green beans is a perfect place to start.

Serves: makes 1 pork roast, serves at least 10
Time: approximately 8 hours

Ingredients:
- 5 lb pork shoulder, fat scored with a sharp knife
- 2 onions, cut into chunks
- 1 cup chicken stock
- Fresh herbs, chopped – rosemary, thyme, oregano, whatever you've got!

Method:
1. Heat some oil in a skillet or fry pan.
2. Place the pork shoulder fat-side down and sear the fat.
3. Sear all sides of the pork until browned.
4. Drizzle some olive oil into the Crock Pot.
5. Place the onion chunks into the pot.
6. Pour the chicken stock over the onions.
7. Place the pork shoulder on top of the onions.
8. Rub the scored pork skin with salt, pepper, and herbs.
9. Place the lid onto the pot and set the temperature to LOW.
10. Cook for 8 hours.
11. Use the leftover liquids to make a gravy if you like! (reduce in a pan and adding more liquid or thickeners if need be).

Beef pot roast

This recipe is much like the previous pork recipe, but this time, beef is the star player. Roast beef is very versatile and makes for a very easy leftovers dinner. This is a great recipe to call on when you want to impress guests!

Serves: makes 1 beef pot roast, serves at least 12
Time: approximately 6 hours

Ingredients:
- 4 lb beef roast, boneless
- 2 onions, cut into chunks
- 6 garlic cloves, skin on
- 1 tbsp Dijon mustard
- 1 cup beef stock
- 1 tsp dried herbs

Method:
1. Heat some oil in a skillet or fry pan.
2. Sear the beef roast on all sides until browned.
3. Drizzle some olive oil into the Crock Pot.
4. Add the onions and garlic to the pot.
5. Mix together the Dijon mustard, beef stock, and herbs.
6. Add the beef to the pot, on top of the onions, rub the beef with salt and pepper.
7. Pour the mustard and stock mixture over the beef.
8. Place the lid onto the pot and set the temperature to HIGH.
9. Cook for 6 hours.
10. Remove the beef from the pot and leave to rest on a board before carving.

Stuffed beef packets

These are little parcels of yumminess. Beef schnitzel is wrapped around a filling of feta cheese, ricotta cheese, spinach, pine nuts, and olives. Despite being very easy to prepare, these packets are very impressive.

Serves: 6
Time: approximately 4 hours

Ingredients:
- 6 slices beef schnitzel
- 4 ounces feta cheese, cut into small chunks
- 1 cup ricotta cheese
- 1 cup baby spinach, chopped
- 18 black olives, chopped
- 3 tbsp pine nuts
- 3 Wooden skewers, cut in half

Method:
1. In a small bowl, mix together the feta cheese, ricotta cheese, spinach, olives, pine nuts, salt, and pepper.
2. Take each piece of beef schnitzel, lay it on a board, and place a dollop of cheese mixture into the middle.
3. Gather the sides of the schnitzel around the filling and tightly wrap.
4. Secure the packet with one of the skewer halves.
5. Sprinkle the tops of the packets with salt and pepper.
6. Drizzle some olive oil into the Crock Pot and set the temperature to HIGH.
7. Place the beef packets into the Crock Pot.
8. Cook for 4 hours.
9. Serve while hot, with a side of relish or Keto-friendly sauce such as garlic mayonnaise!

Paprika drumsticks

Cook a batch of these drumsticks next time you are going to a Summer barbeque, or simply feel like something quick and tasty for dinner. These are so delicious cold from the fridge the next day, so make a few more!

Serves: makes 10 drumsticks
Time: approximately 4 hours

Ingredients:
- 10 chicken drumsticks
- 2 tsp smoky paprika
- 2 eggs, lightly beaten
- ¼ cup ground almond

Method:
1. Mix together the paprika, ground almond, salt, and pepper and spread onto a plate
2. Prepare the chicken drumsticks by dipping them in the beaten egg, then rolling them in the paprika/almond mixture
3. Drizzle some olive oil into the Crock Pot
4. Place the chicken drumsticks into the pot and set the temperature to HIGH
5. Cook for 4 hours
6. Serve hot or cold, with a few fresh salads!

Pork chops with mushrooms and onion

Tender pork chops with creamy mushrooms and onion, served with a side of greens (of course!). A perfect option for a mid-week dinner with just enough decadence to get you through the rest of the week. Use any mushrooms you like; I choose a mixture.

Serves: 4 – 6 (makes 6 pork chops)
Time: approximately 4 hours

Ingredients:
- 6 pork chops
- 4 garlic cloves, finely chopped
- 1 large onion, finely chopped
- 1 tsp mixed dried herbs
- 2 cups chopped mushrooms – a mixture of button, brown, and Portobello is nice!
- 1 cup heavy cream

Method:
1. Rub the pork chops with olive oil, salt, and pepper.
2. Heat some olive oil in fry pan.
3. Add the garlic, onion, and mushrooms to the pot, sauté until soft.
4. Add the cream to the pan and simmer until slightly reduced.
5. Drizzle some olive oil into the Crock Pot.
6. Add the pork chops to the Crock Pot and pour the cream and mushroom mixture over the top.
7. Sprinkle with mixed dried herbs, salt, and pepper.
8. Place the lid onto the pot and set the time to HIGH.
9. Cook for 4 hours.
10. Serve hot, with a spoonful of creamy mushroom sauce over the top!

Slow cooker leek and sausage bake

This is a perfectly over-the-top dish. Tasty sausages mingle with soft leeks and zucchini, with a topping of not one but two kinds of cheeses. Use your favorite Keto-friendly sausages. I like to use pure beef sausages for this recipe, but chicken sausages would be incredible too!

Serves: 6 – 8
Time: approximately 4 hours

Ingredients:
- 6 sausages
- 2 leeks, washed and sliced
- 3 garlic cloves, finely chopped
- ½ cup cream
- 1 cup baby spinach
- 1 cup cream cheese
- 1 egg
- 1 cup grated mozzarella
- Small handful fresh parsley, chopped

Method:
1. Drizzle some olive oil into the Crock Pot.
2. Place the chopped leeks and garlic into the pot.
3. Place the sausages on top of the leeks.
4. Pour the cream over the sausages and leeks and sprinkle with salt and pepper.
5. In a small bowl, mix together the egg, cream cheese, mozzarella, and parsley.
6. Spread the cheese mixture over the sausages and leeks.
7. Place the lid onto the Crock Pot and set the temperature to HIGH.
8. Cook for 4 hours.
9. Serve with a crispy side salad!

Slow cooked leg of lamb

The meat section ends with the classic leg of lamb. The meat is dressed in a delicate combination of flavors such as mustard, red wine, and rosemary. Serve with vegetables, then devour the cold leftover meat the next day!

Serves: makes 1 leg of lamb, at least 8 servings
Time: approximately 10 hours

Ingredients:
- 4 lb leg of lamb, bone in
- 6 garlic cloves, skin off, cut in half
- 2 tbsp Dijon mustard
- ¾ cup red wine
- 1 cup lamb or beef stock
- 1 large sprig fresh rosemary broken into pieces

Method:
1. Heat some oil in a skillet or fry pan.
2. Sear the leg of lamb on all sides in the hot pan.
3. Take the lamb out of the pan and set aside.
4. Pour the red wine and stock into the pan and simmer until slightly reduced then turn the heat off.
5. Drizzle some olive oil into the Crock Pot.
6. Rub the lamb with olive oil, salt, and pepper.
7. With a sharp knife, make 12 incisions on the top of the lamb and push the garlic clove halves and a small piece of fresh rosemary into each incision.
8. Rub the top of the lamb with the mustard.
9. Place the lamb into the Crock Pot and pour the wine and stock mixture over the top of the lamb.
10. Place the lid onto the pot and set the temperature to LOW.
11. Cook for 10 hours.
12. Remove from the Crock Pot and leave to rest for 30 minutes before carving and serving.

One pot creamy mushrooms and steak

Creamy mushrooms and steak – what a mouth-watering combination! Instead of having to stand over a hot, spitting fry pan and a bubbling pot of creamy sauce...make life easier and throw it all into the Crock Pot! The steak comes out soft and tender, (as opposed to charred as you might expect from a skillet or fry pan).

Serves: 4
Time: approximately 3 hours

Ingredients:
- 4 steaks (chuck steak is my favorite for this dish)
- 3 garlic cloves, finely chopped
- 2 cups chopped mixed mushrooms, (white, brown, Swiss)
- 1 cup heavy cream
- ½ beef stock cube dissolved in ¼ cup water (gives lots of extra flavor!)

Method:
1. Rub the steak with olive oil and sprinkle with salt and pepper.
2. Drizzle some olive oil into the Crock Pot.
3. Add the garlic, mushrooms, cream, stock cube mixture, salt, and pepper to the pot, stir to combine.
4. Add the steaks to the pot.
5. Place the lid onto the pot and set the temperature to HIGH.
6. Cook for 3 hours.
7. Serve the steak with a generous serving of creamy mushroom sauce!

Lemongrass and basil chicken thighs

I have lemongrass growing in my garden and the smell is just incredible! You can find lemongrass paste in the supermarket if you don't have fresh lemongrass on hand. The basil in this recipe really lifts the chicken, and creates a lovely fragrance. The coconut cream offers a small amount of moisture and a binding agent to gently combine the lemongrass and basil.

Serves: 3 - 5
Time: approximately 4 hours

Ingredients:
- 6 chicken thighs, boneless, skin on
- 3 garlic cloves, finely chopped
- 2 tbsp crushed lemongrass (fresh or jarred)
- Small handful fresh basil, roughly chopped
- 1/3 cup coconut cream

Method:
1. Drizzle some olive oil into the Crock Pot.
2. Add the chicken, garlic, lemongrass, basil, coconut cream, salt, and pepper to the pot, stir to combine.
3. Place the lid onto the pot and set the temperature to HIGH.
4. Cook for 4 hours.
5. Serve the chicken thighs with a general spoonful of lemongrass, basil, and coconut sauce!

Seafood

Seafood provides lots of nutrition to your diet. Omega 3's and protein are among the many reasons to choose fish and seafood for dinner. Fish and seafood doesn't require as much cooking time in the Crock Pot, so some of these recipes are much quicker than other meat-based recipes. You can use fresh or frozen seafood for many of these dishes.

Fish and tomato stew

This is a very versatile dish, as you can add any extras you like. I like to add black olives and capers sometimes! Use any fresh white fish you can find.

Serves: 4
Time: approximately 4 hours

Ingredients:
- 4 tomatoes, chopped
- 2 cups fish stock
- 5 garlic cloves, finely chopped
- 1 tsp ground cumin
- 1 tsp ground chili
- 1 tsp ground coriander
- 3 large white fish fillets, cut into chunks
- Handful of fresh parsley, chopped

Method:
1. Drizzle some olive oil into the Crock Pot.
2. Add the tinned tomatoes, fish stock, garlic, cumin, chili, coriander, fish, salt, and pepper, stir to combine.
3. Place the lid onto the pot and set the temperature to HIGH.
4. Cook for 4 hours.
5. Serve the stew while hot, with a generous sprinkling of fresh parsley!

Salmon cake

This salmon cake is a great choice for a light dinner or lunch, or a decadent breakfast. Hot smoked salmon fillets work really well in this dish, or you can simply use smoked salmon strips.

Serves: 4 – 6
Time: approximately 4 hours

Ingredients:
- 4 eggs, lightly beaten
- 3 tbsp heavy cream
- 1 cup baby spinach, roughly chopped
- 2 ounces smoked salmon strips, or 1 large fillet of hot smoked salmon, roughly chopped or flaked
- Handful of fresh coriander, roughly chopped

Method:
1. Drizzle some olive oil into the Crock Pot.
2. Place the beaten egg, cream, spinach, salmon, salt, and pepper into the pot and gently stir to combine.
3. Place the lid onto the pot and set the temperature to LOW.
4. Cook for 4 hours.
5. Serve with a generous sprinkling of fresh coriander!

Lemon-butter fish

Tender white fish with lemony butter – it's so incredibly simple! Sometimes the best dishes are the least complicated ones, as the gorgeous ingredients speak for themselves. Serve with fresh greens.

Serves: 6
Time: approximately 5 hours

Ingredients:
- 6 fillets of fresh white fish
- 2 ounces butter, soft but not melted
- 2 garlic cloves, crushed
- 1 lemon
- Handful of fresh parsley, finely chopped

Method:
1. In a small bowl, combine the butter, garlic, zest of one lemon, chopped parsley, salt and pepper.
2. Drizzle some olive oil into the Crock Pot.
3. Place the fish fillets into the Crock Pot and sprinkle with salt and pepper.
4. Place a dollop of lemon butter onto each fish fillet and gently spread it out.
5. Place the lid onto the Crock Pot and set the temperature to LOW.
6. Cook for 5 hours.
7. Serve each fish fillet with a generous spoonful of melted lemon butter from the bottom of the Crock Pot, and a small squeeze of lemon juice over the top!

Creamy seafood chowder

I couldn't NOT add a creamy seafood chowder recipe! This recipe is very rich so a small serving is just enough to satisfy you (and your guests).

Serves: 6
Time: approximately 5 hours

Ingredients:
- 5 garlic cloves, crushed
- 1 small onion, finely chopped
- 1 cup prawns, (frozen is fine, thaw first)
- 1 cup shrimp, (frozen is fine, thaw first)
- 1 cup white fish, chopped into small chunks
- 2 cups full-fat cream
- 1 cup dry white wine
- Handful of fresh parsley, finely chopped

Method:
1. Drizzle some olive oil into the Crock Pot.
2. Add the garlic, onion, prawns, shrimp, white fish, cream, wine, salt, and pepper into the Crock Pot, stir to combine.
3. Place the lid onto the pot and set the temperature to LOW.
4. Cook for 5 hours.
5. Serve while hot, with a sprinkling of fresh parsley!

Salmon and garlic greens

In my opinion, fresh salmon doesn't need a lot of help to be absolutely delicious. This dish combines fresh salmon fillets, greens, and lovely garlic to create a light and elegant dish.

Serves: 4
Time: approximately 3 hours

Ingredients:
- 4 salmon fillets, skin on
- 4 garlic cloves, crushed
- ½ a head of broccoli, cut into florets
- 2 cups frozen green beans

Method:
1. Drizzle some olive oil into the Crock Pot.
2. Place the salmon fillets, (skin-side down) into the pot and sprinkle them with salt and pepper.
3. Place the broccoli, beans, and garlic on top of the salmon, sprinkle the veggies with salt and pepper.
4. Drizzle some more olive oil over top of the veggies and fish.
5. Place the lid onto the pot and set the temperature to HIGH.
6. Cook for 3 hours.
7. Serve immediately!

Prawn and sausage Crock Pot casserole

Prawns and sausage go together very well, especially when slow cooked with spices, herbs, and tomato. I like to use spicy sausage such as chorizo, but you can use any kind of sausage you like!

Serves: 6
Time: approximately 6 hours

Ingredients:
- 1 ½ cups frozen prawns, (thawed)
- 3 sausages, chopped into chunks
- 5 garlic cloves, crushed
- 1 small onion, finely chopped
- 4 tomatoes, chopped
- 1 tsp mixed dried herbs
- 2 tsp mixed dried spices – coriander, cumin, chili (choose your favorites)

Method:
1. Drizzle some olive oil into the Crock Pot.
2. Place the prawns, sausages, garlic, onion, tinned tomatoes, herbs, spices, salt, and pepper into the pot and stir to combine.
3. Place the lid onto the pot and set the temperature to LOW.
4. Cook for 6 hours.
5. Serve while hot, with a sprinkling of fresh herbs such as coriander and parsley!

Coconut fish curry

This curry has a beautiful golden color thanks to the ground turmeric and yellow curry paste. Choose any fresh white fish you can find, and make sure to use full-fat coconut milk.

Serves: 4 – 6
Time: approximately 4 hours

Ingredients:
- 4 large fillets of fresh white fish, cut into chunks
- 4 garlic cloves, crushed
- 1 small onion, finely chopped
- 1 tsp ground turmeric
- 2 tbsp yellow curry paste
- 2 cups fish stock
- 2 cans full-fat coconut milk
- 1 lime
- Fresh coriander, roughly chopped

Method:
1. Drizzle some olive oil into the Crock Pot.
2. Add the garlic, onion, turmeric, curry paste, fish, stock, coconut milk, salt, and pepper to the pot, stir to combine.
3. Place the lid onto the pot and set the temperature to HIGH.
4. Cook for 4 hours.
5. Serve while hot, with a small squeeze of fresh lime juice and fresh coriander!

Fish and bacon soup

Salty bacon adds an extra dimension to this creamy fish soup. Serve with a small squeeze of fresh lemon juice, and a sprinkling of freshly chopped red chili if you like a bit of heat!

Serves: 6
Time: approximately 4 hours

Ingredients:
- 5 slices streaky bacon, chopped
- 4 fillets of fresh white fish, chopped into chunks
- 5 garlic cloves, crushed
- 4 cups fish stock
- 1 cup crème fraiche

Method:
1. Drizzle some olive oil into the Crock Pot.
2. Add the bacon, fish, garlic, stock, salt, and pepper to the pot, stir to combine.
3. Place the lid onto the pot and set the temperature to HIGH.
4. Cook for 4 hours.
5. Remove the lid and stir the crème fraiche into the soup.
6. Serve with an extra dollop of crème fraiche and some freshly chopped herbs!

Mozzarella shrimp parcels

Look, I love any recipe which includes "packet" or "parcel" in the description! So, I had to include my amazing shrimp parcels. These are fantastic to serve as a starter or nibble at a party, or simply to snack on before dinner during the week.

Serves: makes 12 parcels
Time: approximately 3 hours

Ingredients:
- 2 cups frozen shrimp (thawed)
- 12 slices streaky bacon, cut in half
- 2 cups grated mozzarella cheese
- Large bunch of Kale, washed and hard stalks removed
- 12 small skewers, (or 6 long ones, cut in half)

Method:
1. Cut the kale into 12 large pieces – I usually just cut 6 large kale leaves in half, (they need to be large enough to be used as wraps).
2. On a large board, lay out the kale halves.
3. Lay 2 bacon half slices on the kale.
4. Place a small handful of shrimp on top of the bacon.
5. Place a small handful of grated mozzarella on top of the shrimp.
6. Sprinkle with salt and pepper.
7. Wrap the parcels up tightly by folding the sides up, then folding the top and bottom up, and use a skewer to secure them.
8. Drizzle some olive oil into the Crock Pot.
9. Place the parcels into the pot.
10. Place the lid onto the pot and set the temperature to HIGH.
11. Cook for 3 hours.
12. Heat some olive oil into a frying pan.
13. Take the parcels out of the Crock Pot once cooked and transfer them to the hot oil to cook on both sides to create a crisp and golden outer.
14. Serve with your choice of sauces and dips!

Slow cooked coconut lime mussels

If you like mussels, you will love this dish. Creamy coconut, zingy lime, and delicious mussels will entice you to eat the whole lot!

Serves: 4
Time: approximately 2 ½ hours

Ingredients:
- 16 fresh mussels
- 4 garlic cloves
- 1 ½ cup full-fat coconut milk
- ½ red chili, finely chopped
- 1 lime
- ½ cup fish stock
- Handful of fresh coriander, chopped

Method:
1. Drizzle some olive oil into the Crock Pot.
2. Add the garlic, coconut milk, chili, fish stock, salt, pepper, and juice of one lime to the pot, stir to combine.
3. Place the lid onto the pot and set the temperature to HIGH.
4. Cook for 2 hours.
5. Remove the lid, place the mussels into the liquid and place the lid back onto the pot.
6. Cook for about 20 minutes, or until the mussels open.
7. Serve while hot, with a generous serving of coconut and lime sauce over the top, and a big handful of fresh coriander!

Calamari, prawn, and shrimp "pasta" sauce

This sauce is fantastic on top of Keto-friendly pasta such as spiralized zucchini. You can also serve it as a soup or stew, but because it is rather rich, I think it works best with fresh veggies. You can use frozen seafood, just thaw it before cooking!

Serves: makes a large portion of sauce, enough for about 5 pasta servings
Time: approximately 3 hours

Ingredients:
- 1 cup calamari
- 1 cup prawns
- 1 cup shrimp
- 6 garlic cloves, crushed
- 4 tomatoes, chopped
- 1 tsp dried mixed herbs
- 1 tbsp balsamic vinegar

Method:
1. Drizzle some olive oil into the Crock Pot.
2. Add the calamari, prawns, shrimp, garlic, tinned tomatoes, mixed herbs, balsamic vinegar, salt, and pepper, stir to combine.
3. Place the lid onto the pot and set the temperature to HIGH.
4. Cook for 3 hours.
5. Serve with zucchini noodles or a side of fresh veggies!

Slow cooked whole fish with ginger and soy

There's nothing more impressive than a whole fish, served on a platter with fresh garnishes and a few simple veggies to serve it with. This recipe uses Asian-inspired flavors such as ginger and soy. Use any fresh, whole white fish you can find.

Serves: makes one whole fish, about 4 servings
Time: approximately 2 hours

Ingredients:
- 1 fresh, whole fish
- 4 garlic cloves, crushed
- 2 tbsp grated fresh ginger
- 4 tbsp soy sauce

Method:
1. Score the fish with a sharp knife by cutting diagonal lines through the skin.
2. Rub the fish with olive oil.
3. Sprinkle the fish with sea salt and pepper.
4. Sprinkle the grated ginger onto the fish and rub it into the scores.
5. Drizzle some olive oil into the Crock Pot.
6. Place the fish into the pot.
7. Pour the soy sauce over top of the fish.
8. Place the lid onto the pot and set the temperature to HIGH.
9. Cook for 2 hours.
10. Serve immediately! Garnish with fresh green herbs to give a pop of color.

Slow cooked sesame prawns

Mmmm, tender prawns and the nutty taste of sesame oil and sesame seeds. I add lots of chili to this recipe, because I love the heat, but you can leave the chili out or just add a little bit! Serve over cauliflower rice.

Serves: 4
Time: approximately 2 hours

Ingredients:
- 3 cups large prawns, (if using frozen, thaw first)
- 4 garlic cloves, crushed
- 1 tbsp sesame oil
- 2 tbsp toasted sesame seeds
- ½ red chili, finely chopped
- ½ cup fish stock

Method:
1. Drizzle the sesame oil into the Crock Pot.
2. Add the prawns, garlic, sesame seeds, chili, and fish stock to the pot, stir well to coat the prawns.
3. Place the lid onto the pot and set the temperature to HIGH.
4. Cook for 2 hours.
5. Serve while hot, with fresh herbs and cauliflower rice!

Crock Pot tuna steaks

Tuna steaks are not as commonly-used as salmon, but they are delicious! This recipe is very simple, as I want the tuna flavor to come through, rather than being masked by other strong flavors.

Serves: 4
Time: approximately 3 hours

Ingredients:
- 4 tuna steaks
- 3 garlic cloves, crushed
- 1 lemon, sliced into 8 slices
- ½ cup white wine

Method:
1. Reduce the white wine in a pot by simmering until the strong alcoholic smell is cooked off.
2. Rub the tuna steaks with olive oil, and sprinkle with salt and pepper.
3. Place the tuna steaks into the Crock Pot.
4. Sprinkle the crushed garlic on top of the tuna steaks.
5. Place 2 lemon slices on top of each tuna steak.
6. Pour the reduced wine into the pot.
7. Secure the lid onto the pot and set the temperature to HIGH.
8. Cook for 3 hours.
9. Serve with a drizzle of leftover liquid from the pot, and a side of crispy greens!

Salmon with leeks and cream

Leeks are one of the best vegetables to use in the Crock Pot. The subtle onion flavor and buttery softness add a true sophistication to any dish. This dish is ideal for special occasions, as the rich, creamy sauce and oily salmon just begs for an audience!

Serves: 4
Time: approximately 4 hours

Ingredients:
- 4 fresh salmon fillets
- One leek, finely sliced
- 1 cup heavy cream
- ½ cup white wine

Method:
1. Pour the cream and wine into a pot, bring to a simmer and reduce until slightly thickened.
2. Rub the salmon fillets with olive oil, and sprinkle with salt and pepper.
3. Drizzle some olive oil into the Crock Pot.
4. Add the leeks to the pot and sprinkle with salt and pepper.
5. Place the salmon fillets on top of the leeks.
6. Pour the reduced cream and wine mixture into the pot.
7. Place the lid onto the pot and set the temperature to LOW.
8. Cook for 4 hours.
9. Serve the salmon with a generous serving of leeks and creamy sauce!

Desserts

If you thought you had to say goodbye to desserts while on the Ketogenic diet...good news! There are many Keto-friendly desserts to enjoy, and I've chosen a selection of my ultimate favorites. A few of these recipes use stevia to add Keto-friendly sweetness. You can find stevia in most supermarkets, or simply order some online! Oh and by the way...there are lots of chocolate recipes in this section, so I'm crossing my fingers that you're as much of a chocoholic as me!

Keto coconut hot chocolate

Making hot chocolate in the Crock Pot is easy and fun! This recipe is rich, creamy, and not too sweet. Make sure you buy dark chocolate with the highest cocoa percentage you can find. This recipe only contains a small amount of chocolate, but the rest of the chocolaty-ness is made up by cocoa.

Serves: 8
Time: approximately 4 hours

Ingredients:
- 5 cups full-fat coconut milk
- 2 cups heavy cream
- 1 tsp vanilla extract
- 1/3 cup cocoa powder
- 3 ounces dark chocolate, roughly chopped
- ½ tsp cinnamon
- Few drops of stevia to taste

Method:
1. Add the coconut milk, cream, vanilla extract, cocoa powder, chocolate, cinnamon, and stevia to the Crock Pot and stir to combine.
2. Place the lid onto the Crock Pot and set the temperature to HIGH.
3. Cook for 4 hours, whisking every 45 minutes.
4. Taste the hot chocolate and if you prefer more sweetness, add a few more drops of stevia.
5. Enjoy with a dollop of whipped cream on top!

Ambrosia

Ambrosia is a pillowy, fluffy, creamy mixture of yogurt, cream and berries. Topped with coconut, almond, and dark chocolate...you'll melt into a puddle of joy! The topping is prepared in the Crock Pot, but the base is easy to whip up in a bowl in 5 minutes.

Serves: 8 – 10
Time: approximately 4 hours

Ingredients:

- 1 cup unsweetened shredded coconut
- ¾ cup slivered almonds
- 3 ounces dark chocolate (high cocoa percentage), roughly chopped
- 1/3 cup pumpkin seeds
- 2 ounces salted butter
- 1 tsp cinnamon
- 2 cups heavy cream
- 2 cups full-fat Greek yogurt
- 1 cup fresh berries – strawberries and raspberries are best

Method:

1. Place the shredded coconut, slivered almonds, dark chocolate, pumpkin seeds, butter, and cinnamon into the Crock Pot.
2. Place the lid onto the pot and set the temperature to HIGH.
3. Cook for 3 hours, stirring every 45 minutes to combine the chocolate and butter as it melts.
4. Remove the mixture from the Crock Pot, place in a bowl, and leave to cool.
5. In a large bowl, whip the cream until softly whipped.
6. Stir the yoghurt through the cream.
7. Chop the strawberries into small pieces and add to the cream mixture, along with the other berries you are using, fold through.
8. Sprinkle the cooled coconut mixture over the cream mixture.
9. Serve in bowls with an extra grating of dark chocolate on top!

Dark chocolate and peppermint pots

These velvety pots are smooth, rich, and surprisingly refreshing thanks to the peppermint essence. I like to make these at Christmas time, as they have a lovely festive feel. Serve with a fresh mint leaf on top of each pot, just to jazz it up a bit!

Serves: makes 6 pots
Time: approximately 3 hours

Ingredients:
- 2 ½ cups heavy cream
- 3 ounces dark chocolate, melted in the microwave
- 4 egg yolks, lightly beaten with a fork
- Few drops of stevia
- Few drops of peppermint essence to taste

Method:
1. Mix together the beaten egg yolks, cream, stevia, melted chocolate and peppermint essence in a medium-sized bowl.
2. Prepare the pots by greasing 6 ramekins with butter.
3. Pour the chocolate mixture into the pots, evenly.
4. Place the pots into the Crock Pot and very carefully pour hot water into the pot, (around the pots so it doesn't get into the chocolate mixture!) until it reaches just below half way up the pots.
5. Place the lid onto the Crock Pot and set the temperature to HIGH.
6. Cook for 2 hours.
7. Take the pots out of the Crock Pot and leave to cool and set.
8. Serve with a fresh mint leaf and a dollop of whipped cream on top!

Creamy vanilla custard

This creamy vanilla custard can be served alone, or with a few strawberries sprinkled on top. This custard is very creamy and rich so a small serving goes a long way!

Serves: 8
Time: approximately 3 hours

Ingredients:
- 3 cups full-fat cream
- 4 egg yolks, lightly beaten
- 2 tsp vanilla extract
- Few drops of stevia

Method:
1. In a medium-sized bowl, whisk together the cream, egg yolks, vanilla extract, and stevia.
2. Pour the mixture into a heat-proof dish (one that fits into the Crock Pot!).
3. Place the dish into the Crock Pot.
4. Pour enough hot water into the pot, around the dish, so that it reaches half way up the sides of the dish.
5. Place the lid onto the pot and set the temperature to HIGH.
6. Cook for 3 hours.
7. Serve hot or cold!

Coconut, chocolate, and almond truffle bake

Gooey balls of coconut, chocolate, and almonds baked together to form a soft, decadent dessert perfect for Keto-friendly special occasions. It's sort of like a sweet dessert casserole...

Serves: 6 – 8
Time: approximately 4 hours

Ingredients:
- 3 ounces butter, melted
- 3 ounces dark chocolate, melted
- 1 cup ground almonds
- 1 cup desiccated coconut
- 3 tbsp unsweetened cocoa powder
- 2 tsp vanilla extract
- 1 cup heavy cream
- A few extra squares of dark chocolate, grated
- ¼ cup toasted almonds, chopped

Method:
1. In a large bowl, mix together the melted butter, chocolate, ground almonds, coconut, cocoa powder, and vanilla extract.
2. Roll the mixture into balls.
3. Grease a heat-proof dish (make sure it fits in the Crock Pot).
4. Place the balls into the dish.
5. Place the lid onto the pot and set the temperature to LOW.
6. Cook for 4 hours.
7. Leave the truffle dish to cool until warm.
8. Whip the cream until it is soft and pillowy.
9. Spread the cream over the truffle dish and sprinkle the grated chocolate and chopped toasted almonds over the top.
10. Serve immediately!

Peanut butter, chocolate and pecan cupcakes

These cupcakes are inspired by the delicious peanut butter cups we all know and love. Topped with chopped toasted pecans, the sweet and salty combination is irresistible! Peanut butter is fine on Keto as long as you only have small amounts, and this recipe gives you just enough peanutty goodness to satisfy you, but it won't upset your Ketosis. A great holiday treat for Keto dieters.

Serves: makes 14 chocolate cups
Time: approximately 4 hours

Ingredients:
- 14 paper cupcake cases
- 1 cup smooth peanut butter
- 2 ounces butter
- 2 tsp vanilla extract
- 5 ounces dark chocolate
- 2 tbsp coconut oil
- 2 eggs, lightly beaten
- 1 cup ground almonds
- 1 tsp baking powder
- 1 tsp cinnamon
- 10 pecan nuts, toasted and finely chopped

Method:
1. Melt together the dark chocolate and coconut oil in the microwave, stir to combine and set aside.
2. Place the peanut butter and butter into a medium-sized bowl, microwave for 30 seconds at a time until the butter has just melted.
3. Stir together the peanut butter and butter until combined and smooth.
4. Stir the vanilla extract into the peanut butter mixture.
5. In a small bowl, mix together the ground almonds, eggs, baking powder, and cinnamon.
6. Pour the melted chocolate and coconut oil evenly into the 14 paper cases.
7. Spoon half of the almond/egg mixture evenly into the cases, on top of the chocolate and press down slightly.
8. Spoon the peanut butter mixture into the cases, on top of the almond/egg mixture.

9. Spoon the remaining almond/egg mixture into the cases.
10. Sprinkle the chopped pecans on top of each cupcake.
11. Very carefully place the filled cases into the Crock Pot, if they don't all fit, use a rack (so there are 2 levels of cakes).
12. Place the lid onto the pot and set the temperature to HIGH.
13. Cook for 4 hours.
14. Remove the cakes from the pot and leave to cool.
15. Serve warm, with a dollop of whipped cream!

Vanilla and strawberry cheesecake

Cheesecake! I would eat cheesecake everyday if I could. This recipe is Keto-friendly, and absolutely divine. Serve this at your next dinner party; even if your guests are carb eaters, they will love it!

Serves: 8
Time: approximately 6 hours

Ingredients:

Base:
- 2 ounces butter, melted
- 1 cup ground hazelnuts
- ½ cup desiccated coconut
- 2 tsp vanilla extract
- 1 tsp cinnamon

Filling:
- 2 cups cream cheese
- 2 eggs, lightly beaten
- 1 cup sour cream
- 2 tsp vanilla extract
- 8 large strawberries, chopped

Method:
1. Prepare the base: in a medium-sized bowl, combine the melted butter, hazelnuts, coconut, vanilla, and cinnamon.
2. Press the base into a greased heat-proof dish (make sure it fits into the Crock Pot).
3. In a large bowl, place the cream cheese, eggs, sour cream, and vanilla extract, beat with electric egg beaters until thick and combined.
4. Fold the strawberries through the cream cheese mixture.
5. Pour the cream cheese mixture into the dish, on top of the base, spread out until smooth.
6. Place the dish into the Crock Pot and pour enough hot water around the dish so that it comes half way up the side of the dish.
7. Place the lid onto the pot and set the temperature to LOW.
8. Cook for 6 hours until just set but slightly wobbly.
9. Allow to cool slightly before placing in the fridge until cold.
10. Serve with a dollop of whipped cream!

Coffee creams with toasted seed crumble topping

Cooked in ramekins, these coffee-flavored custards are a wonderful way to end a meal. The crunchy seed topping adds a great texture and gentle nutty flavor.

Serves: makes 6 ramekins
Time: approximately 4 hours

Ingredients:
- 2 cups heavy cream
- 3 egg yolks, lightly beaten
- 1 tsp vanilla extract
- 3 tbsp strong espresso coffee (or 3tsp instant coffee dissolved in 3tbsp boiling water)
- ½ cup mixed seeds – sesame seeds, pumpkin seeds, chia seeds, sunflower seeds,
- 1 tsp cinnamon
- 1 tbsp coconut oil

Method:
1. Heat the coconut oil in a small fry pan until melted.
2. Add the mixed seeds, cinnamon, and a pinch of salt, toss in the oil and heat until toasted and golden, place into a small bowl and set aside.
3. In a medium-sized bowl, whisk together the cream, egg yolks, vanilla, and coffee.
4. Pour the cream/coffee mixture into the ramekins.
5. Place the ramekins into the Crock Pot.
6. Pour enough hot water into the pot to reach half way up the ramekins.
7. Place the lid onto the pot and set the temperature to LOW.
8. Cook for 4 hours.
9. Remove the ramekins from the Crock Pot and leave to cool slightly on the bench.
10. Sprinkle the seed mixture over the top of each custard before serving.

Lemon cheesecake

Yes, another cheesecake recipe. I couldn't help myself! Although fruits are not usually permitted on the Keto diet, a grating of lemon zest and a small amount of lemon juice is absolutely fine!

Serves: 8 – 10
Time: approximately 6 hours

Ingredients:
- 2 ounces butter, melted
- 1 cup pecans, finely ground in the food processor
- 1 tsp cinnamon
- 2 cups cream cheese
- 1 cup sour cream
- 2 eggs, lightly beaten
- 1 lemon
- Few drops of stevia
- 1 cup heavy cream

Method:
1. Mix together the melted butter, ground pecans, and cinnamon until it forms a wet, sand-like texture.
2. Press the butter/pecan mixture into a greased, heat-proof dish (make sure it fits in the Crock Pot) and set aside.
3. Place the cream cheese, eggs, sour cream, stevia, zest and juice of one lemon into a large bowl, beat with electric egg beaters until combined and smooth.
4. Pour the cream cheese mixture into the dish, on top of the base, smooth it out so that the top of the cheesecake is even.
5. Place the dish into the Crock Pot and pour enough hot water into the pot so that it reaches half way up the side of the dish.
6. Place the lid onto the pot and set the temperature to LOW.
7. Cook for 6 hours.
8. Set the cheesecake on the bench to cool and set.
9. Whip the cream until soft and pillowy, and spread over the cheesecake before serving.

Macadamia fudge truffles

These fudge truffles are soft, decadent, nutty, and chocolatey...make a big batch of them and gift them to your Keto friends for birthdays and special occasions! Slow cooking the mixture creates a very gooey texture.

Serves: makes about 25 small truffles
Time: approximately 4 hours

Ingredients:
- 1 cup roasted macadamia nuts, finely chopped
- ½ cup ground almonds
- 2 ounces butter, melted
- 5 ounces dark chocolate, melted
- 1 tsp vanilla extract
- 1 egg, lightly beaten

Method:
1. Place the macadamia nuts, almonds, melted butter, melted chocolate, vanilla, and egg into a large bowl, stir until combined.
2. Grease the bottom of the Crock Pot by rubbing with butter.
3. Place the mixture into the Crock Pot and press down.
4. Place the lid onto the pot and set the temperature to LOW.
5. Cook for 4 hours.
6. Remove the lid, turn the cooker off, and allow the mixture to cool until just warm.
7. Take a teaspoon and scoop the mixture out of the pot, and roll into balls until all mixture has been used.
8. Place the balls on a plate or in a container and refrigerate to harden slightly.
9. If you like, you can roll the balls in unsweetened cocoa powder to finish!
10. Store the truffle balls in the fridge.

Chocolate covered bacon cupcakes

I know, this recipe title might seem completely mad at first! But I promise - salty bacon pieces, dark chocolate, and a nutty cake mixture make for a beautiful combination.

Serves: makes 10 cupcakes
Time: approximately 3 hours

Ingredients:

- 10 paper cupcake cases
- 5 slices streaky bacon, cut into small pieces, fried in a pan until crispy
- 5 ounces dark chocolate, melted
- 1 cup ground hazelnuts
- 1 tsp baking powder
- 2 eggs, lightly beaten
- ½ cup full-fat Greek yogurt
- 1 tsp vanilla extract

Method:

1. In a small bowl, mix together the fried bacon pieces and melted chocolate, set aside.
2. In a medium-sized bowl, mix together the ground hazelnuts, baking powder, eggs, yoghurt, vanilla, and a pinch of salt.
3. Spoon the hazelnut mixture into the cupcake cases.
4. Spoon the chocolate and bacon mixture on top of the hazelnut mixture.
5. Place the cupcake cases into the Crock Pot (careful not to spill!).
6. Place the lid onto the Crock Pot and set the temperature to HIGH.
7. Cook for 3 hours.
8. Remove the cupcakes from the pot and leave to cool on the bench before storing serving.
9. Serve with whipped cream!

Chocolate, berry, and macadamia layered jars

I use little jars for this recipe, but you can use ramekins if you don't have mini jars. These desserts have a cream cheese surprise in the center, among chocolate, berries, and macadamia nuts.

Serves: makes 6 jars (or ramekins)
Time: approximately 6 hours

Ingredients:
- 5 ounces dark chocolate, melted
- ½ cup mixed berries, (fresh) – any berries you like
- 3/4 cup toasted macadamia nuts, chopped
- 7 ounces cream cheese
- ½ cup heavy cream
- 1 tsp vanilla extract

Method:
1. In a medium-sized bowl, whisk together the cream cheese, cream, and vanilla extract.
2. Spoon a small amount of melted chocolate into each jar or ramekin (only use half of the chocolate).
3. Place a few berries on top of the chocolate (use half of the berries).
4. Sprinkle some toasted macadamias onto the berries (use half of the nuts).
5. Spoon a dollop of the cream cheese mixture into the ramekin (use all of the cream cheese mixture).
6. Place another layer of chocolate, berries, and macadamia nuts on top of the cream cheese mixture.
7. Place the jars into the Crock Pot and pour enough hot water into the pot so that it reaches half way up the sides of the jars.
8. Place the lid onto the pot and set the temperature to LOW.
9. Cook for 6 hours.
10. Remove the jars and leave them to cool and set on the bench for about 2 hours before serving.

Salty-sweet almond butter and chocolate sauce

This sauce can be poured over any of the desserts in this section for a decadent upgrade. A small amount goes a long way, so be sparing with your servings!

Serves: makes 1 jar of sauce
Time: approximately 4 hours

Ingredients:
- 1 cup almond butter
- 2 ounces salted butter
- 1 ounce dark chocolate
- ½ tsp sea salt
- Few drops of stevia

Method:
1. Place the almond butter, butter, dark chocolate, sea salt, and stevia to the Crock Pot.
2. Place the lid onto the pot and set the temperature to LOW.
3. Cook for 4 hours, stirring every 30 minutes to combine the butter and chocolate as they melt.
4. Pour into a jar and leave to cool before storing in the fridge.

Coconut squares with blueberry glaze

Coconut and blueberry are a great combination! A small square will satisfy your dessert craving, without ruining your Keto diet efforts. You can swap the blueberries for other kinds of berries if you wish!

Serves: about 20 small squares
Time: approximately 3 hours

Ingredients:
- 2 cups desiccated coconut
- 1 ounce butter, melted
- 3 ounces cream cheese
- 1 egg, lightly beaten
- ½ tsp baking powder
- 2 tsp vanilla extract
- 1 cup frozen berries

Method:
1. In a large bowl, place the coconut, butter, cream cheese, egg, baking powder, and vanilla extract, beat with a wooden spoon until combined and smooth.
2. Grease a heat-proof dish (make sure it fits inside the Crock Pot) with butter.
3. Spread the coconut mixture into the dish.
4. Place the blueberries into a small bowl and defrost in the microwave until they resemble a thick sauce.
5. Spread the blueberries over the coconut mixture.
6. Place the dish into the crock pot and pour enough hot water into the pot so that it reaches half way up the dish.
7. Place the lid onto the pot and set the temperature to HIGH.
8. Cook for 3 hours.
9. Remove the dish from the pot and leave to cool on the bench before slicing into small squares.

Chocolate and blackberry cheesecake sauce

I just had to slip in another cheesecake-based recipe (I can't resist), so I've added this delicious cheesecake sauce! This can be served over many of the recipes in this section, or simply drizzled over a few berries for a light and yummy Keto dessert.

Serves: makes 1 jar of sauce
Time: approximately 6 hours

Ingredients:
- ¾ lb cream cheese
- ½ cup heavy cream
- 1 ½ ounces butter
- 3 ounces dark chocolate
- ½ cup fresh blackberries, chopped
- 1 tsp vanilla extract
- Few drops of stevia (optional, depending on how sweet you prefer your sauce)

Method:
1. Place the cream cheese, cream, butter, dark chocolate, blackberries, vanilla, and stevia into the Crock Pot.
2. Place the lid onto the pot and set the temperature to LOW.
3. Cook for 6 hours, stirring every 30 minutes to combine the butter and chocolate as it melts.
4. Pour into a jar and leave to cool before storing in the fridge.
5. Have a spoonful here and there to curb your sweet cravings! Or pour over Keto desserts or berries!

Conclusion

Did you find some new favorite recipes to make in your Crock Pot or slow cooker? I hope so. Remember, you can adjust and change these recipes to suit your budget, tastes, and required servings.

How is your Keto experience turning out? I hope you are feeling those amazing benefits we talked about earlier in the book! Don't beat yourself up if you are struggling, or have struggled, to stick to the Keto diet at first! It can take time to get used to, and there's no shame in having a few slip ups. Remember to eat enough to keep you full, satisfied, and full of energy. Even if you can't see the results of the Keto diet yet from the outside, rest assured that your insides are thanking you for all of the fresh nutrients!

If you have just bought your Crock Pot, I bet you are loving it already! And if you're a long-time Crock Pot fan, I know you're sticking by your trusty on-pot kitchen hero.

So long for now, and thanks for coming along on this Keto Crock Pot adventure!

Made in the USA
San Bernardino, CA
01 November 2018